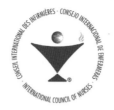

International Council of Nurses
Advanced Nursing Practice

MADREAN SCHOBER, MSN, NP-C, FAANP
Nurse Practitioner
International Healthcare Consultant
Schober Consulting
Indianapolis, Indiana, USA

FADWA A. AFFARA, MA, MSc, RN, SCM
International Nurse Consultant
Education and Regulatory Policy
Edinburgh, Scotland

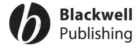

Blackwell
Publishing

© 2006 International Council of Nurses (ICN)

Blackwell Publishing Ltd,
Editorial offices:
Blackwell Publishing Ltd, 9600 Garsington Road, Oxford OX4 2DQ, UK
  Tel: +44 (0)1865 776868
Blackwell Publishing Inc., 350 Main Street, Malden, MA 02148-5020, USA
  Tel: +1 781 388 8250
Blackwell Publishing Asia Pty Ltd, 550 Swanston Street, Carlton, Victoria 3053, Australia
  Tel: +61 (0)3 8359 1011

The right of the Author to be identified as the Author of this Work has been asserted
in accordance with the Copyright, Designs and Patents Act 1988.

First published 2006 by Blackwell Publishing Ltd

2 2007

ISBN 978-14051-2533-8

Library of Congress Cataloging-in-Publication Data
Schober, Madrean.
    International Council of Nurses : advanced nursing practice / Madrean
  Schober, Fadwa A. Affara.
      p. ; cm.
    Includes bibliographical references and index.
    ISBN-13: 978-1-4051-2533-8 (pbk. : alk. paper)
    ISBN-10: 1-4051-2533-0 (pbk. : alk. paper)
    1. Nurse Practitioners. 2. Primary care (Medicine) I. Affara, Fadwa
  A. II. International Council of Nurses. III. Title. IV. Title: Advanced
  nursing practice.
    [DNLM: 1. Nurse Practitioners. 2. Nurse's Role. 3. Nursing Care.
  WY 128 S363i 2006]
  RT82.8.S25 2006
  610.7306′92–dc22

                                                                2006006420

A catalogue record for this title is available from the British Library

Set in 10/12.5pt TimesNRMT
by Graphicraft Limited, Hong Kong
Printed and bound in Singapore
by Fabulous Printers Pte Ltd

The publisher's policy is to use permanent paper from mills that operate a sustainable
forestry policy, and which has been manufactured from pulp processed using acid-free and
elementary chlorine-free practices. Furthermore, the publisher ensures that the text paper
and cover board used have met acceptable environmental accreditation standards.

For further information on Blackwell Publishing, visit our website:
www.blackwellnursing.com

Contents

Foreword

Today, nurses across the world are at the forefront of innovation and development in health care. Advanced nursing practice is one of the dynamic and exciting developments we have seen evolve over the past few decades as a result. This book offers the reader an insight into the inception of advanced nursing practice, describing the numerous developments occurring in all regions. In documenting the many opportunities and challenges raised through health systems reform, the book offers a range of solutions and frameworks and maps out an agenda for the future. In short, this text provides a valuable insight into a significant component of nursing practice in the 21st century.

To be effective, advanced nursing practice must be anchored within the local health system and tailored to meet the needs of the client or population group. This means that globally, advanced nursing practice, while sharing many similarities, also looks different in different parts of the world. This is reflected and illustrated through the authors' own extensive international experience, and the evidence they have gathered from key informants and practitioners in the field through dialogue and questionnaires.

The various chapters tackle significant issues in the development of advanced practice. Every chapter draws extensively on the rich data available and offers a range of illustrations on how nurses and nursing have responded to the needs of often underserved populations or communities across the world. The use of vignettes, coupled with the various models and frameworks, provides readers with a range of approaches rather than a single prescriptive solution, and gives grounded and practical illustrations of the issues faced by nurses at the forefront of these developments.

Front-line nurses are not alone in developing innovative responses. Educators, policy makers, regulators, the public, other disciplines and researchers all have a role to play. Indeed, without the support and contribution of these stakeholders, the scope of advanced nursing practice is limited and progress in its development and implementation delayed.

Affara and Schober have done the profession an important service by drawing together such a rich resource into a single text. Advanced nursing practice has seen great progress over the past decades, but the journey is far from over. Nurses, regulators, educators and policy makers from across the world will continue to develop this work to meet the needs of the public. As nursing practice evolves and changes, advanced nursing practice has an important role to play. This role will continue to develop as part and parcel of wider health systems reform and this text offers insights into that future.

Hiroko Minami
President
International Council of Nurses

Preface

For us who nurse, our Nursing is a thing, which, unless we are making progress every year, every month, every day . . . we are going back.

Florence Nightingale, 1872[1]

Countries in membership with the International Council of Nurses (ICN) are reporting that changes in health care have given impetus to the development of innovative models of care and new roles for nurses. However, these shifts in health systems have created uncertainty over boundaries of practice, appropriate models of care, legal status, professional accountability and responsibility, and questions about the nature and level of education required. Nurses and key stakeholders are searching for information and guidance to help shape new roles to match the current realities and needs of their practice settings.

The purpose of this book is to examine what is happening in the field of advanced nursing practice internationally. It deals with themes that are important to the development and acceptance of advanced practice nurses as a valid and necessary part of the health workforce. In exploring recurrent issues and emerging international trends, the authors discuss the distinctive nature of advanced nursing practice, role definition, practice development, education, regulation and research. In addition, the book draws on successful experiences and discusses strategies for managing change when implementing sustainable advanced nursing practice roles, in a way that will be helpful to those seeking, or are currently engaged in workforce development.

The authors draw on their international experience especially that obtained through their close association with the initiation and development of ICN's International Nurse Practitioner/Advanced Practice Nursing Network. Key informants, a review of the literature and other unpublished sources complement experiences of the authors. Key informants have been used as, apart from in a few countries, little has been documented about what is happening in this area. The key informants have been selected on the basis that they are formal and informal leaders, influential leaders or experts who know what is going on in one or more aspects of advanced nursing practice in their country.

---

[1] Nightingale, F. (1872). *For us who nurse.*

The 49 key informants from 24 countries represent experienced clinicians, nurse regulators, nursing association staff, educators, researchers and nurses holding governmental positions. All the key informants were asked to complete a questionnaire which can be found in Appendix 1.

Across the spectrum of persons consulted, experiences examined and literature reviewed, similar issues and questions recurred, and need to be examined and addressed if advanced nursing practice is to take hold. These have been succinctly summarised in a WHO document on promoting the development of advanced practice in the Eastern Mediterranean Region (EMR) in this way:

- Agreement that the role is needed
- Agreement on how the role will enhance health care services
- Support (human and financial) for appropriate educational standards
- Agreement on inter- and intra-professional issues
- Consensus on competencies required for the role
- Clarity on legal and ethical considerations
- Methods for introducing advanced practice nurse roles
- Procedures for title protection
- Conformity in standard treatment guidelines
- Recruitment and retention policies for students, faculty and clinicians (WHO-EMR, in press).[2]

Through this book, the authors hope to contribute to the debate around the areas identified by WHO-EMR. Concepts, strategies, and problematic areas in relation to the nature of advanced nursing, role development, regulation, education and research are explored. Vignettes, illustrations and examples drawn from actual experience are used to depict how nurses working in very different situations and settings are moving towards the advanced practice roles. Tools such as environmental scans, questions for debate and guidelines, as well as additional resources, are provided to assist readers who are interested in promoting an appropriate place for advanced nursing practice in modern health care systems.

The authors found there is no ideal model of advanced nursing practice emerging, and no one system that would suit nursing in all its variability worldwide. Major difficulties and a lack of clarity exist around the identity, standards, role in the health system and education of advanced nursing practice. Accordingly, this publication will be useful as a guide intended to assist in the development and implementation of advanced nursing practice while taking account of situational factors in individual countries, the profession's stage of development in that context and the profession's particular goals.

It is hoped that this book proves useful to nurses and others, whether in direct practice, education, involved with regulatory bodies or professional nursing

---

[2] World Health Organization, Regional Office for the Eastern Mediterranean Region. (In press). *Advanced nursing practice guidelines*, EMRO Technical Publications Series 29, Cairo.

organisations seeking to initiate role development, strengthen its acceptance within health services, set up educational programmes, or reinforce the current advanced practice role in their country, and those for whom the service is intended.

It is envisaged that it can be used by:

- Professional groups (national nurses' associations, professional regulatory bodies, policy makers, educators) seeking to inform key groups of the role, potential impact and benefits of having advanced practice nurses
- Professional groups directly involved in developing the role or evaluating and/or reforming existing systems, policies or practices
- Educators, administrators and decision makers in institutions providing the education who need further understanding of this aspect of professional role
- Policy makers involved in health workforce planning and in establishing health workforce regulatory policies, and members of the public interested in promoting advanced nursing practice services in their communities.

What you will find in this book

Chapter one surveys the current state of advanced nursing practice internationally and discusses how international agreement was arrived at over the definition of an advanced practice nurse.

Chapter two examines the nature of advanced nursing practice and the characteristics of the role. Issues that surround titling, scope of practice, competencies, and a number of controversial areas such as prescribing and diagnosing are discussed. Tools for developing a scope of practice are included.

Chapter three on role and practice development suggests a process for carrying out an environmental scan. It proposes using a stakeholder analysis which looks at how groups of people affecting the emergence and development of advanced nursing practice might react, and a SWOT analysis to identify key factors that may impact on the advanced nursing practice role in terms of the strengths, weaknesses, opportunities and threats existing in the environment. Strategies for implementing and sustaining the role are suggested and vignettes are used to illustrate the ways that advanced nursing practice is emerging in diverse settings. The vignettes are intended as a resource for those seeking to persuade key decision-makers to support advanced nursing practice development.

Chapter four focuses on regulatory and legislative matters. It places advanced nursing practice regulation within the larger arena of professional regulation. Models and frameworks are suggested to guide in the formulation of adequate and supportive regulatory/legislative framework for advanced practice nurses. A process for exploring the regulatory environment is suggested.

Chapter five discusses education for advanced nursing practice. Curriculum development, faculty preparation and managing the clinical practicum are some of the areas explored. Sample course descriptions, preceptor guidelines and evaluation forms are provided in the appendices. Vignettes are used to describe different routes adopted to prepare advanced practice nurses in diverse settings.

Chapter six starts with a short discussion on the theoretical perspective of advanced nursing practice, and suggests the type of research and environment that would assist in supporting advanced nursing practice knowledge and practice development. An international research agenda for advanced nursing practice is identified. Ways to enhance knowledge and skills are discussed.

Chapter seven envisages future prospects for advanced nursing practice in areas such as: primary health care; managing chronic conditions and offering home care services; in the growing telehealth areas; and as nurse entrepreneurs. The authors conclude by identifying four critical challenges that need serious attention if advanced practice nurses are to evolve and find a place in national health systems that use their potential for the full benefit of individuals, families and communities.

Fadwa A. Affara, *MA, MSc, RN, SCM*
International Nurse Consultant: Education and Regulatory Policy

Madrean Schober, *MSN, NP-C, FAANP*
Nurse Practitioner
International Healthcare Consultant

Acknowledgements

The authors are eternally grateful to the contribution made by the key informants. They gave generously of their time by completing a lengthy questionnaire, and answering our follow-up queries. We appreciate their honesty and frankness in sharing successes and failures, hopes and aspirations. Their contributions have infinitely enriched our personal knowledge and experience, and what we had learned from the literature on this subject. A Japanese proverb tells us: 'There are no national frontiers to learning.' The key informants have proved that to us many times.

Australia
Mollie Burley
Lecturer, Centre for Multi-Discipline Studies,
Monash University of Rural Health
Victoria

Trisha Dunning
Professor and Director, Department of Endocrinology and Diabetes Nursing Research
St Vincent Hospital and the University of Melbourne
Fitzroy, Victoria

Anna Green
ICU Liaison Nurse Practitioner,
Western Hospital
Footscray, Victoria

Desley Hegney
Professor of Rural and Remote Area Nursing,
Universities of Queensland and Southern Toowoomba, Queensland

Bahrain
Amina Matooq
Head Post-Basic Cardiac Nursing, College of Health Sciences
Manama

Botswana
Onalenna Seito
Head of Department of Family Practice, Trainer of Family Nurse Practitioners
Institute of Health Sciences
Gabarone

Canada
Sandra Easson-Bruno
Clinical Nurse Specialist
President, Canadian Association of Advanced Practice Nurses
International Nurse Practitioner/Advanced Practice Nurse Network, Education
and Practice Sub-Group
Barrie, Ontario

Linda Jones
Primary Health Care Nurse Practitioner
Ottawa, Ontario

Cynthia Struthers
Acute Care Nurse Practitioner
Former Associate Chief of Nursing Practice
Treasurer of Canadian Association of Advanced Practice Nurses
International Nurse Practitioner/Advanced Practice Nurse Network, Research
Sub-Group
Mississauga, Ontario

Louise Sweatman
Director, Regulatory Policy
Canadian Nurses Association
Ottawa

Denmark
Bente Sivertsen
Chief Professional Nursing Officer, Danish Nurses Organization
Copenhagen

Hong Kong
Susie Lum
Senior Executive Manager (Nursing)
Hospital Authority
Hong Kong

Tso Shing-yuk, Alice
General Manager in Nursing
Hospital Authority
Kowloon Cluster Hospitals
Hong Kong

Iceland
Gudbjorg Gudmundsdottir
Clinical Nurse Specialist
Landspitali University Hospital
Reykjavik

Ireland
Kathleen MacLellan
Head of Professional Development
National Council for the Professional Development of Nursing and Midwifery
Dublin

Japan
Kiyoka Nozue
Professor and Certified Nurse Specialist
Faculty of Nursing and Medical Care
Keio University
Tokyo

Shiori Usami
Professor and Certified Nurse Specialist
Department of Nursing
Kumamoto University
School of Health Sciences
Kumamoto

Jordan
Da'ad Shokeh
Registrar
Jordan Nursing Council
Amman

Macau
Florence Van Lat Kio
Director and Professor
Kiang Wu College of Nursing of Macau
Vice-President of The Nurses Association of Macau
Macau

Yin Lei
Director
School of Health Sciences
Macau Polytechnic Institute

The Netherlands
Kathleen Sullivan-Mulder
Professor

Nurse Practitioner Education
Leeuwarden

Petrie F. Roodbol
Head of Nursing
University Medical Center Groningen
Institute of Education
Groningen

New Zealand
Marion Clark
Chief Education Officer
Nursing Council of New Zealand
Wellington

Alison Dixon
Head of School
School of Nursing
Otago Polytechnic
Dunedin

Merian Litchfield
Independent Consultant
Wellington

Jean Ross
Principal Lecturer
School of Nursing
Otago Polytechnic
Dunedin

Susanne Trim
Professional Nursing Adviser
New Zealand Nurses' Organisation
Wellington

Pakistan
Yasmin Amarsi
Professor and Dean
School of Nursing
The Aga Khan University
Karachi

Philippines
Geogracia Valderrama
School of Health Sciences
College of Nursing

Mapua Institute of Technology
Vice Chairman of the Nursing Specialty Certification Council
Manila

Singapore
Siu Yin Lee
Director of Nursing
National University Hospital
Singapore

South Africa
Nelouise Geyer
Deputy Director Professional Matters
Democratic Nursing Organisation of South Africa
Pretoria

Sudan
Awatif Ahmed Osman
Dean
Faculty of Nursing Sciences
Academy of Medical Sciences and Technology
Khartoum

Switzerland
Sabina De Geest
Professor and Lecturer
Institute of Nursing Science
University of Basel
Basel

Lyn Lindpaintner
Lecturer
Institute of Nursing Science
University of Basel
Basel

Rebecca Spirig
Associate Professor of Nursing and Chair of the Division of Clinical Nursing
Science
Institute of Nursing Science
University Hospital of Basel
Basel

Sweden
Elsie-Britt Hallman
Lecturer

School of Life Sciences
University of Skovde

Ella Danielson
Associate Professor
The Sahlgrenska Academy at Göteborg University
Institute of Nursing
Göteborg

Elisabet Zetterström
Lecturer
Department of Health Sciences
Mid-Sweden University
Östersund

Taiwan
Mei-Nah Hwang
Director
Bureau of Nursing and Health Services Development
Taipei

Thailand
Prathana Langkarpint
Nurse Researcher and Educator
Payap University
Chiang Mai

Somchit Hanucharurnkul
Professor and Chairman of Doctoral Program in Nursing
Ramathibodi School of Nursing
Mahidol University
Bangkok

United Kingdom
Sue Cross
Associate Director of Primary Care Nursing for Bedfordshire and Hertfordshire
Clifton

Morag White
Nurse Practitioner
General Practice
Northern Ireland

Cherry Cullen
Nurse Practitioner in Primary Health Care
Aylesford Medical Centre
Aylesford

Katrina Maclaine
Royal College of Nursing Nurse Practitioner Adviser
NP Team Leader
London South Bank University
London

United States
Mary Brown
Assistant Professor of Clinical Nursing
University of Texas Health Science Center at Houston
Houston

Joanne V. Hickey
Professor
Division Head, Acute and Critical Care
Director, Acute Care Nurse Practitioner and Critical Care Clinical Nurse
Specialist Programs
Director/Coordinator for the new Doctor of Nursing Practice (DNP)
University of Texas Health Science Center at Houston
Houston

Rosemary Goodyear
Nurse Consultant Associates
Faculty Associate, University of San Diego
Independent Consultant
International Nurse Practitioner/Advanced Practice Nurse Network, Chair of
Core Group
San Diego

Lorna Schumann
Director of the Family Nurse Practitioner Program
Intercollegiate College of Nursing
Washington State University

Joyce Pulcini
Associate Professor
William F. Connell School of Nursing
Boston College

Lenore Kolljeski Resick
Professor
Director Nurse-Managed Wellness Centers
Interim Director Family Nurse Practitioner Program
Duquesne University School of Nursing
Pittsburgh

Chapter 1
Introduction

Advanced nursing practice: a growing presence

Halfan Mahler during his term as Director General of the World Health Organization (WHO) declared to the WHO Executive Board:

> *If the millions of nurses in a thousand places articulate the same ideas and convictions about primary heath care, and come together as one force, then they could act as a powerhouse for change (WHO, 1985).*

These words continue to resonate today for nurses around the globe as they harness their experience, energy, knowledge and commitment to improve the quality of care through adapting and expanding practice. For instance, we learn that in many of the island countries in the Western Pacific:

> *nurses diagnose, and treat patients on a regular basis; dispense medication; provide all maternal and child health care including deliveries; provide some dental care, perform minor surgical procedures, keep statistics (in Fiji nurses even do the census); and provide community outreach services (Abou Youssef et al., 1997, p. 9).*

During the 1990s, the International Council of Nurses (ICN) monitored the growing presence of advanced nursing practice roles as countries reformed health systems, and sought innovative health care options in efforts to keep up with demands, trends and economic constraints. There appeared to be a better acceptance of new nursing roles and practice models, which included initiatives such as nurse prescribing of medications and treatments; diagnosis and ordering of laboratory tests; and referral and admitting rights.

Schober (2002) identified a number of other factors contributing to a greater demand for an expanded scope for nurses. These included overcoming access barriers to primary health care (PHC); rising demands for specialised nursing services; the growth in home health care nursing where more clients needed complex care; the desire for professional advancement; and escalating disease rates worldwide.

The New Zealand Ministry of Health (NZMOH), recognising the existence of increasing numbers of highly educated nurses with advanced clinical and leadership competencies, believed this untapped potential could be released for greater use in health care if nurses are facilitated to:

- Use their knowledge and skills more effectively
- Pioneer innovative services provision
- Enhance the access to, and quality of, primary health care
- Contribute positively to health gain (NZMOH, 2002, p. 4).

As more evidence emerges suggesting that optimising the nursing contribution to health care through expanding their role is an effective strategy for improving health services (WHO-EMRO, 2001; WHO, 2002; NZMOH, 2002; Buchan & Calman, 2004), authorities are more prepared to seek solutions that include this option. Mounting costs, limited fiscal resources, increasing health challenges, and rising public expectations for health care have encouraged governments to accept that adequate coverage and access to the health services are more important than who provides them. In 2002 WHO commented:

> *Shortages in many countries of health care professionals mean that new approaches to organizing teams of staff are required; traditional role boundaries may be a hindrance. Skills that have been the province of physicians may become common practice for nurses, while some nursing roles may be taken over by health care assistants (WHO, 2002).*

Also, as Schober & McKay (2004) point out, recent models of practice tend to be more collaborative when there is 'mutual recognition of discrete and shared competencies and respect for the interests and roles and responsibilities of all participants' (p. 8). The trend to partnership and collaboration in practice is compatible with the scopes of practice in the new roles nurses are beginning to carve out.

Advanced nursing practice: patterns of development

This section gives an overview of what the authors have uncovered about the existence of advanced nursing practice or similar type roles around the world. The authors, aware that there are developments going on this area that are not documented or not accessible for various reasons, have drawn heavily on the information provided by the key informants who have been generous and patient with explaining how advanced nursing is evolving in their situation.

In a fluid international context deciding what constitutes advanced practice is not easy, especially as international understanding of the role differs and consensus on title does not exist. Therefore, for the purposes of charting the presence of advanced nursing practice in this chapter, the authors have included what is reported and considered by the key informants to fall under the broad category of advanced practice as they understand it.

The expanded role of the nurse is not a modern phenomenon. Keeling and Bigbee (2005) trace the roots of advanced nursing practice in the USA to the 19th century. The term specialist began to be employed in the early years of the twentieth century as more postgraduate courses in specific areas of practice became available. Nurse anaesthetists, nurse midwives and psychiatric clinical nurse specialists (CNS) led the way, but the growth of hospitals in the 1940s and the development of medical specialties and technologies stimulated the evolution of CNS. These nurses were judged to practise at a higher level of specialisation than that already present in nursing (Schober, 2005), and are the precursors of the modern CNS. In the 1960s, nurse practitioners (NP) were created in the USA to provide primary health care services to populations with unmet needs, and promote community-based continuity of care. As this group began to push the boundaries of nursing practice even further, they faced greater challenges from other groups, especially physicians who considered NPs to be encroaching on their domain of practice.

Advanced practice nurse (APN), an umbrella term coined in the USA to cover the types of nurses working in diverse advanced roles, is defined by the American Nurses Association as 'a registered nurse (RN) who has met advanced educational and clinical practice requirements beyond the 2–4 years of basic nursing education required of all RNs' (ANA, 1993). By 1993, the ANA estimated there were about 140 000 APNs, which in the USA context included clinical nurse specialists (CNS), nurse practitioners (NP), nurse anaesthetists (NA) and nurse midwives (NM).

Nurse midwives and nurse anaesthetists began to appear in Korea in the 1950s. By the 1980s they were joined by community health nurse practitioners (CHNP) carrying a wide range of responsibilities (Kim, 2003; Schober & Affara, 2001). This latter category, created to serve isolated rural areas and fishing villages, was recognised through legislation after sustained political action by nurses. Nurses were able to support their proposals with data documenting that nurses, in contrast to other health professions, were more successful in providing efficient services to these populations (Cho & Kashka, 2004). Later, home care nursing was added to the advanced practice categories, and in 2000 the title was legally changed from *special field nurse* to *advanced practice nurse*. Now ten types of APNs are recognised through certification (Kim, 2003).

In Japan the first master of nursing programme aimed to prepare nurse researchers, but as medicine diversified and specialised it became clear that nursing had to develop practice to fit this development. The first CNS graduate programme was in psychiatric and mental health nursing and graduated its first students in 1986 (key informant, personal communication). Certification came later when the Japanese Nurses' Association (JNA), in partnership with the Japanese Association for Nursing Programmes in University (JANPU), initiated a postgraduate course in 1994 for certified nurse specialists. In addition to completing a masters degree in nursing-related studies and earning a specified number of credits in an area of specialisation as defined by the JANPU, to become a CNS a nurse must be certified by JNA (ICN Credentialing Forum, 2004a). By

2005, Japan had 139 practising CNS. Initially certification was available in psychiatric and mental health and oncology, but it now can be obtained in community, critical care, geriatric, paediatric, maternal and chronic adult nursing. The functions of the CNS lie in practice, consultation, coordination, ethical coordination, education and research (key informant, personal communication).

Another JNA initiative was to create the certified expert nurse (CEN) in 1966, a non-university-based qualification obtained after taking a JNA accredited programme. (ICN Credentialing Forum, 2002; JNA News 2002). There were over 1 741 CENs by 2005, practising in 17 areas such as emergency nursing, wound /ostomy/continence care, critical care, hospice, cancer and chemotherapy, diabetes, infection control, and infertility nursing.

Since 2003 the JNA certification scheme has been evaluated, and has demonstrated that the posting of CNS in emergency and oncology settings is valued, and has a positive influence on health care costs. However, there has been a reluctance to recognise the special contribution of CNS through giving appropriate reimbursement, and there was a tendency to compensate them through promotion to a head nurse position. In a breakthrough in 2005, a special allowance is now being paid to all CNS and CENs working in national hospitals (ICN Credentialing Forum, 2005b).

Taiwan employed the first CNS in cardiac surgery in 1994. While CNS quickly spread to other areas, legislation recognising the role in the health system was to come later in 2000 (Chen, 2005). However, standards of education, scope of practice, and credentialing processes remained undefined until 2004 when agreement on scope of practice, regulations for education, and credentialing processes was reached. In addition, the Department of Health has established an NP advisory committee to oversee national development of this role (Chao, 2005).

The Hospital Authority of Hong Kong introduced the nurse specialist post in 1994 hoping that it would motivate nurses to remain in clinical practice. The implementation of the role without regulatory oversights resulted in an uneven development of the clinical, education and research components, with research being the aspect given the lowest priority (Chang & Wong, 2001). The development of the APN in Hong Kong is related to the move of basic nursing education to the tertiary education setting, and efforts by the Hong Kong Hospital Authority to introduce a new grading structure designed to improve the clinical focus of nurses (key informant, personal communication). The role is slowly evolving as Hong Kong begins to integrate its first graduates from masters programmes (Loke & Wong, 2005).

In the same region, Singapore signalled its intent to embark on the advanced practice route by launching a masters degree in nursing in 2003. The advanced practice role has been legitimised by amending the Nurses and Midwives Bill in 2005, and removing the *nurse specialist* as a category recognised in the Bill, and introducing the *advanced practice nurse*. The Bill also provides for an expanded role and defines required educational qualifications. Annual renewal of the APN practice certificate and continuing education will be conditions for practice (Singapore Ministry of Health, 2005).

While nurse anaesthetists were recognised in 1988, it took a further ten years to have the advanced practice role accepted more generally within the Thai health system. As academic nursing is well established, Thailand is well placed to provide a masters education for this role. The Thai Nursing Council conducted the first certification examination for advanced practice nurses in 2004 (key informant, personal communication).

Advanced nursing practice roles are beginning to emerge in certain countries in Europe, shaped as in other parts of the world by the contexts in which they operate. In the United Kingdom nurses described as demonstrating a *higher-level practice* (United Kingdom Central Council [UKCC], 1999) have moved into settings ranging from general practice and ambulatory care to the chronic and acute care specialties (Royal College of Nursing, [RCN], 2002 revised 2005). White (2001) writes that the emergence of the NP is an acknowledgment of the inadequacy of past medically dominated approaches to health care, and a reaction to the physician shortage in primary care. The United Kingdom has not found it easy to agree on a concept of advanced practice resulting in confusion over scope, titles and education for the role (Woods, 2000; Castledine, 2003).

In 1995, the UK's regulatory body established a standard for what it calls *specialist practice.* However after a recent consultation, the Nursing and Midwifery Council (NMC) recognised that with role expansion and the growing number of NPs and consultant nurses

> *a significant amount of health care is provided by nurses practising independently, managing case loads of patients and clients in a variety of hospital and community settings . . . There has been common agreement that the standards for the level of specialist practice are no longer robust enough to prepare practitioners for these new roles (NMC, 2005, p. 7).*

The consultation indicated there is widespread support for advanced practice regulation with preference for the title *advanced nurse practitioner*. The NMC proposes legal recognition of nurses practising beyond specialist practice (NMC, 2005).

Lorensen *et al.* (1998) describe the emergence in Nordic countries of a role similar to the CNS in the USA as hospitals employed nurses with graduate education to promote research and develop expert clinical roles. Most CNS have developed in fields associated with medical problems such as diabetes, hypertension and psychiatric disorders. Iceland traces the development of CNS to the return of nurses from the USA with masters qualifications. At first Icelandic hospitals were not ready to accept APNs, but universities welcomed them as faculty. Once the government agreed to license nurse specialists in 2003, hospitals became more willing to employ nurses in specialist posts (key informant, personal communication).

The NP type role has been slower to emerge in Nordic countries probably because the supply of physicians was adequate (Lorensen *et al.*, 1998). However, Sweden is now exploring the use of NPs as a strategy to improve access to primary health care (key informant, personal communication), and in providing care to the elderly in the community (Danielson, 2003). Educational programmes have been established for these two areas. The primary health care authorities in Skaraborg worked with the University of Skovde to develop a model and educational programme that met the requirements of the National Board of Health and Welfare and community primary health care needs as well as preparation as an APN. The first students were enrolled in 2003. The challenge has been to introduce a new role and function that fits the Swedish health system and is acceptable to all stake holders (key informant, personal communication). In doing so they have been able to negotiate the following definition:

> *An Advanced Nurse Practitioner in Primary Health Care is a registered Nurse with special education as a district nurse with the right to prescribe certain drugs, and with a post graduate education that enables [the advanced nurse practitioner] an increased and deepened competence to be independently responsible for medical decisions, diagnosing, prescribing of drugs and treatment of health problems within a certain area of health care (key informant, 2005).*

Currently the Danish Nurses Organisation (DNO) is seeking national approval for a definition for specialty and advanced nursing practice. However, educational programmes that have the potential to prepare nurses for advanced practice are in place. Aarhus University offers masters courses in nursing science and clinical nursing and access to PhD degrees in nursing. Post-registration specialty education is offered by Danish centres of higher education. These programmes are regulated by the National Board of Health and developed in collaboration with the Board of Nurses' specialty and higher education (ICN Credentialing Forum, 2005a).

The advanced nursing practice role was implemented in hospitals in the Netherlands in 1997 as an answer to a shortage of physicians. Its introduction was opportune as the government was seeking to tackle some of the structural health system difficulties by introducing a readjustment of the scopes of practice of doctors and nurses. Nurse practitioners first appeared in a large hospital where dynamic nursing leadership and supportive management policies allowed for the creation of posts and access to education opportunities (key informants, personal communication).

Advanced nursing practice is a recent development in Switzerland and is being led by the Institute of Nursing Science (INS) at the University of Basel, the first institute in Switzerland affiliated to a university. The INS invested in advanced nursing practice through its masters degree in nursing science, their research programmes, and clinical field development activities (key informant, personal communication). The effort to introduce advanced nursing flies in the face of cost containment measures that favour the introduction of more less-educated nurses into the health workforce in Switzerland. Thus, the impetus to create APN posts is not policy driven, but comes from far-sighted nurse leaders in hospital settings in some cases, and physicians interested in working with nurses with higher level clinical skills in others. Recently there has been more attention on expanded roles for nurses as 'physician assistants'. This seems to be concerned not with strengthening nursing, but to cope with an anticipated physician shortage in primary care (key informant, personal communication). Examining how to expand the role of nurses and other paramedicals to cope with future physician shortages concords with what was described in the Netherlands and fits with recent developments in France.

The pioneers of advanced nursing in Switzerland have expended a great deal of effort in marketing the APN role to all interested parties, including nurses. There is growing acceptance of APNs but this is being done in the absence of a legal, policy and reimbursement framework.

In France, the first signs of interest in advanced nursing practice are beginning to surface. Although French nurses did acquire more autonomy in 1978, they still cannot be a point of entry into the health system. Private practice nurses (*infirmières libérales*) are unable to act without a medical order in delivering professional nursing care. To be reimbursed by the social security, the nursing assessment is prescribed by a physician, and the written care plan must be approved by the social security expert physician. However recently health authorities, realising that the present configuration of the health care workforce will be inadequate to respond to health care demand especially of an ageing population, has started to consider other alternatives, including the creation of APNs. ANFIIDE, the French nurses association, capitalising on this situation, has conducted a public information campaign on the advanced practice option which targeted nurses, authorities and the public (C. Debout, personal communication).

With the passage of the Royal Decree of Nursing Specialties in 2005 in Spain, the General Council of Nursing, which functions both as a regulatory and professional organisation, is developing a certification process for nurse specialists. This is a natural outcome of the 2003 legal framework for health professionals which gave access to professional advancement through a process of continuing education and the progressive development of more advanced competencies. However, it is yet unclear how far these emerging roles will demonstrate the key characteristics of advanced nursing practice (ICN Credentialing Forum, 2005c).

While in remote regions of Australia registered nurses with extended role functions have operated without legal or formal recognition for several decades, the first legally recognised NPs were registered in 2001. Multiple initiatives have been launched over the past few years to explore the use of NPs in different settings (Turner & Keyzer, 2002; Victoria Government of Department of Human Services, 2000; key informants, personal communication). This development was underpinned by efforts on the part of regulators (Gardner *et al.*, 2004) and professional organisations (National Nursing Organizations of Australia [NNOA], 2003) to reach national consensus on definition, scope, education and regulation and deal with inconsistencies and confusion that have followed the state-by-state approach adopted by their federated system (Jamieson & Williams, 2002).

In New Zealand the shift to population-based and PHC services combined with a realisation by the government that nurses do have unexploited potential to provide a greater range of services, ignited interest in introducing NPs into the health workforce (New Zealand Nurses Organization [NZNO], 2000; Nursing Council of New Zealand [NCNZ], 2002; 2004; NZMOH, 2002; key informants, personal communication). As a result legislation and regulatory mechanisms are now in place recognising the NP. Additionally, as Australia and New Zealand are bound by the Trans-Tasman Mutual Recognition Agreement, the two countries have proposed a common set of NP standards and competencies (Gardner *et al.*, 2004).

For over four decades in remote areas, Canada has used registered nurses with advanced preparation to provide a range of health care services including primary care functions normally limited to general or family physicians (Centre for Nursing Studies, 2001; Nurse Practitioner Association of Ontario [NPOA], 2005; key informants, personal communication). The advanced practice role in acute care similar to the CNS was initially introduced in the 1970s and by the late 1980s Canada was also preparing advanced practice nurses to a masters level for acute care practice under different titles (key informants, personal communication). The CNS role in Canada was developed to:

> *enhance or improve nursing care by bringing expert practice to direct patient care at the bedside, expert indirect care to other nurses through role modelling and consultation, and to provide an avenue for those nurses who wished to advance, but remain at the bedside (Fahey-Walsh, 2004, p. 13).*

To overcome a physician shortage in rural and remote areas, the primary health care NP (PHCNP) was introduced in the early 1970s but by the mid 1980s the NP movement came to a halt. A variety of factors, including a greater availability of doctors, no legislative framework or recognition in the career structure and poor public awareness led to fall off in NP development and a discontinuation of the educational programmes until the 1990s (NPAO, 2005).

To complicate the Canadian scene a category of acute care NP (ACNP) has grown alongside the CNS. They are employed largely in acute care facilities to deal with complex health problems requiring more in-depth knowledge of nursing and of specific diseases. While currently educational preparation of PHCNPs varies from a registered nurse diploma with additional education and experience to graduate preparation, the vast majority of ACNPs are educated at the graduate level (Fahey-Walsh, 2004).

Now there is renewed interest in Canada in NPs as cost-effective health care providers, especially in PHC, but each province and territory has pursued different approaches to education, licensure and scope of practice. Over recent years several initiatives have been undertaken to facilitate the emergence of a national approach to advanced nursing practice. In 2002, the Canadian Nurses Association (CNA) developed a national framework for advanced nursing identifying the key elements in the areas related to assumptions, definition and characteristics, competencies, educational preparation, domains of practice, roles and regulation. This was followed by a national dialogue with key stakeholders due to conclude in late 2005. Currently, the government is funding a multiple stakeholder NP initiative to create a pan-Canada framework for facilitating the introduction and permanent integration of NPs into the Canadian health system (CNPI, 2005).

The WHO Eastern Mediterranean Regional Office (WHO-EMRO), aware that advanced nursing practice and nurse prescribing were growing issues in the region, consulted all countries in the region on both issues (WHO-EMRO, 2001). A patchy picture emerges where nurses with advanced practice qualifications, usually obtained from abroad, are constrained by lack of legal, professional and institutional recognition. While nurses may be carrying out advanced tasks, the full expression of the advanced practice role is rarely demonstrated or officially permitted. However, in Iran the Ministry of Health has approved an expansion of nurses' functions in different community settings, and plans are in place to regulate advanced practice (WHO-EMRO, 2001). While Jordan has prepared nurses to the master's level since 1986, there is no official recognition of the advanced practice role. However, in the current strategic plan of the Jordanian Nursing Council (2004), the improvement of education and establishment of regulation for the role are included. Finally, in this region advanced nursing practice is beginning to emerge in the health facilities of the Aga Khan University in Pakistan, mostly as a result of the conditions created by the launching of a masters degree in nursing in 2001 by the School of Nursing, though on the whole there is little understanding of the APN role in the country (key informant, personal communication).

Botswana, in the 1970s, created the family nurse practitioner (FNP) to work in the PHC sector, an important health sector as 70% of the population living in rural areas depend on community-based services for care (Seitio, 2000). Functions undertaken by FNPs include taking a full history, conducting physical examinations, diagnosing, prescribing, ordering diagnostic tests, and acting as resources for other nursing personnel. Emphasis is placed on assessment, diagnosis, management of common diseases, disease prevention and health promotion. While Swaziland had an NP programme which produced 102 NPs, the programme was discontinued and the NP role is not recognised within the system (M.D. Mathunjwa, personal communication). Plans are under way to reintroduce the programme as a postgraduate diploma for nurses who have a Bachelor of Science in Nursing (BSN) degree.

Munjanja *et al.* (2005) do report the emergence of clinically focused master's degrees in Botswana, Nigeria, South Africa, Zambia and Zimbabwe, but there is little available documentation that this has translated into developing an acknowledged advanced nursing practice role in the African region. For instance, the ICN Family Nurse Project found nurses in South Africa undertaking elements of the advanced practice role in primary health care (Schober & Affara, 2001) in the South African health system, but Radebe (2000) noted that they are ill prepared to do so. It is possible that current work to articulate a Charter of Practice by the South African Nursing Council (2004) will stimulate interest in providing a distinctive professional and regulatory framework for APNs in South Africa.

In the Caribbean region, Jamaica is in the process of enacting legislation to register NPs. Delays to the passage of the Act are related to difficulties in deciding what type of structure to set up for administering advanced practice credentialing within the Nursing Council (ICN Credentialing Forum, 2004b). While the Pan-American Health Organization (1999) reports that well-established nursing specialisation programmes exist in certain Latin American countries (Colombia, Chile, Ecuador, Mexico, Panama and Venezuela), at present there is little information to judge if developments in these specialties are driving the emergence of a distinct advanced practice role. Ketefian *et al.* (2001), referring specifically to Brazil, believe that factors such as the need to expand nursing to meet basic health needs, the shortage of nurses and the high ratio of physicians to nurses have contributed to inhibiting progress in the advancement of nursing.

Nurse anaesthetists have been organised internationally since 1989 when 11 national associations formed the International Federation of Nurse Anaesthetists (IFNA). Currently associations from 32 countries are members, representing 40 000 nurse anaesthetists from Africa, Asia, the Caribbean, Europe and North America. IFNA has established international standards for education and practice and a code of ethics, and is an affiliated member of ICN (IFNA, 2004).

After this tour around the globe in search of advanced nursing practice in all its different manifestations and stages of development, the next section discusses the findings of an ICN survey, and subsequent actions of the ICN to create a mechanism where all the disparate strands of advanced nursing practice come together to discuss, share and develop an international consensus around the core area of the APN role.

Advanced nursing practice: a global picture

In 2000, ICN conducted a preliminary survey of nurse practitioner/advanced practice roles. At that time, ICN while being aware that the advanced practice role was well established in the United States, and increasingly in Australia, Canada, New Zealand and the UK, knew little about developments in the rest of the world. ICN surveyed its membership of 120 national nurses' associations (NNA) and invited those attending the advanced practice session at the ICN International Conference in London in 1999 and the International Nurse Practitioner Conference in the following year to respond (ICN, 2001). Survey results were ready for the launching of the ICN International Nurse Practitioner/Advanced Practice Nursing Network (INP/APNN) at the 8th International Conference of Nurse Practitioners in San Diego in 2000. The network was set up as an international forum where nurse practitioners and advanced practice nurses could share educational, practice, research and regulatory developments.

Questions covered the nature of the presence of an advanced practice role in their country, characteristics, educational preparation, practice rights and the country's regulatory oversight processes. One hundred and nine surveys were returned from 40 countries.

The picture gleaned from the responses was one of a heightened interest in the advanced nursing practice role, but with a lot of uncertainties, ambiguities and gaps. Thirty-three (83%) of the 40 countries reported that, while there is a nursing role requiring education beyond that of a licensed or registered nurse in the country, the level of education for these roles was varied. In 30 (69%) countries formal educational programmes preparing individuals for advanced nursing roles existed, but in only 26 (65%) did the education lead to a recognised qualification such as a degree, diploma or certificate. While 31 (78%) of the countries have some kind of accreditation or approval process in place for the educational programme, accrediting or approval agencies were very different in nature ranging from national nursing boards or councils, departments or ministries of health or education to federations of nursing schools, universities, private accrediting bodies and local government. Thirteen (33%) countries had legislation or some other type of regulatory mechanism for nurse practitioners/advanced practice.

The situation was less certain when it came to the titles in use. Fifteen (36%) of the countries reported having a specific title for advanced roles, some countries had more than one title in use. While nurse practitioner, clinical nurse specialist and nurse specialist were mentioned, a variety of other names were given to this role. Chapter two explores this point further.

Variability was more pronounced when it came to role characteristics. A relatively high number identified that nurses working in the advanced role were involved in planning, implementing and evaluating programmes (73%), provided consultant services to health providers (70%), had research functions (68%), were recognised as one of the first point contacts for clients (68%), and had the authority to refer clients to other professionals (60%). However, claimed role characteristics fell significantly when it involved areas likely to conflict with the traditional role of other health care providers such as having autonomy and independence in practice (55%), the authority to prescribe treatments (38%), the right to diagnose (35%), and the authority to prescribe medicines (25%).

Since ICN started monitoring the advanced practice field through the ICN network, considerable progress has been made worldwide. A survey taken three years later prior to the INP/APNN's third international conference indicated that over 60 countries are currently developing or implementing advanced practice nursing roles. Mounting issues of concern in implementation of advanced nursing roles were for the most part related to the education for, and the evaluation of, competence (Roodbol, 2004).

Definition of the advanced practice nurse

ICN's position on regulation emphasises that clear definitions are fundamental to identifying and placing a profession within the heath care system (Styles & Affara, 1997). These definitions are important because they identify who the health worker is, and define boundaries for practice. Thus definitions can be thought of as shorthand ways to communicate what services to expect from what health worker, and how it will be offered.

To define and guide the work of ICN's INP/APNN it was agreed that reaching consensus on an international definition for the APN was its first priority. Countries struggling with the early stages of role definition and development were particularly eager to have an international definition available to them.

The initial step taken was to draft a working definition of the APN and identify characteristics of the role. These were drawn from analysis of country-specific papers on progress of advanced nursing practice submitted to the network; a review of literature; and the results of the ICN survey. The draft definition, accompanied by a discussion paper and response sheet, was sent to ICN national nurses' associations (NNA), the network subgroups and all its members. All the documents were posted on the web and responses were invited. Twenty-six responses were received from 11 countries and represented opinion from NNAs, regulatory bodies, WHO and individual nurses. The responses tended to come from countries where there was some familiarity with the role.

A high level of agreement was reached that the proposed definition is representative of present and potential roles in the responding countries. The recommended masters degree for entry stimulated most debate, but the argument seemed to reflect the different stages of advanced practice development and availability of educational programmes rather than a fundamental disagreement of the unsuitability of this level of education. Some respondents were not comfortable with the bias of the draft definition which seemed to imply that advanced practice was reserved to primary health care (Duffy, 2002).

A further difficulty arose with respect to the title as the terms APN and NP are used inconsistently and interchangeably both within nations, and from one country to another. Although NP is the title that is most frequently protected and defined, APN is in substantial use. To decide on one term would run counter to network strategy to be inclusive and open to all the variations of the role at this stage of international development. Thus both titles are included in the first ICN definition.[1] In 2002, ICN's Board of Directors approved a definition, which broadens the role beyond primary health care, and recommends rather than stipulates a masters level education. Finally, it is important to note that the definition is not intended to be prescriptive, but was established to facilitate common international understanding and foster unity around this emerging role.

The ICN position is that the nurse practitioner/advanced practice nurse is:

a registered nurse who has acquired the expert knowledge base, complex decision-making skills and clinical competencies for expanded practice, the characteristics of which are shaped by the context and/or country in which s/he is credentialed to practice. A masters degree is recommended for entry level (ICN, 2002).

---

[1] For the purpose of clarity, the authors will use the term APN in general discussion of the developments and issues around this role.

The definition is further expanded by the delineation of characteristics in the domains of education, practice and regulation. These will be discussed in greater detail in Chapter 2.

Conclusion

It is inevitable that as advanced nursing practice evolves around the world, roles associated with its practice will be influenced by the profession's identity and values, the nature of the health care context and socio-political imperatives and current priorities. What emerges from the authors' attempt to make some sense of the patterns emerging, as advanced nursing practice is taken up by more countries, is a picture of confusion and different interpretations as to what is advanced nursing practice. The large number of titles in use, a lack of agreement over the routes and standards of education, and no clear consensus over scope of practice make it difficult to define a clear and distinctive identity for APNs. This uncertainty directs our attention to the need for more rigorous exploration and research of these topics.

Nevertheless, since ICN started to monitor the emergence of advanced nursing practice globally, there appears to be increasing consensus over the usefulness of APNs in a country's health system and greater convergence over role definition, education and regulatory requirements. In defining the APN and identifying the characteristic of this role, ICN has taken the first step towards clarifying the nature of APN practice. A scope of practice definition, standards for regulation and education and APN competencies are being developed at the time of writing, and will serve as a foundation for further dialogue on this issue.

Currently nurses in advanced practice roles are to be found in many health care settings. Nurses, the largest group of health providers in most parts of the world, do have within their grasp a host of opportunities to advance their roles and become core frontline providers of quality, cost-effective health care. However, nurses are no longer willing to accept that contributing to health services in this way remains unacknowledged. There is a growing determination to have these roles officially recognised, regulated and appropriately reimbursed. If advanced nursing practice is acknowledged as a valid part of the health system, and is supported by appropriate education, adequate regulation and career pathways, it has the potential to increase nurses' capacities to work in advanced roles independently and collaboratively in multiple settings.

References

Abou Youssef, E.Y., Bisch, S.A., Hiejnan, S., Hirschfeld, M.J., Land, S., Leenders, F., Manfredi, M., Miller, T.E., Ngcongco, V.N., Salvage, J., Stilwell, B., Tornquist, E. (1997). *Nursing practice around the world.* Geneva: Nursing/Midwifery, Health Systems Development Programme, World Health Organization.

American Nurses Association. (1993). *Nursing facts: Advanced practice nursing: A new age in health care.* Retrieved July 7, 2005 from http://nursingworld.org/readroom/fsadvprc.htm

Buchan, J., Calman, L. (2004). *Skill-mix and policy change in the health workforce: Nurses in advanced practice roles.* OECD Working Paper No 17, Paris, OECD. Retrieved 30 September, 2005 from http://www.oecd.org/dataoecd/30/28/33857785.pdf

Canadian Nurse Practitioner Initiative. (2005). *Frequently asked questions about nurse practitioners.* Retrieved July 9, 2005 from http://www.cnpi.ca/faq.asp

Canadian Nurses Association. (2002). *Advanced nursing practice. A national framework.* Ottawa: Author.

Castledine G. (2003). The development of advanced nursing practice in the UK. In P. McGee, G. Castledine (Eds) *Advanced nursing practice*, 2nd Edition, pp. 8–16. Oxford: Blackwell Publishing.

Centre for Nursing Studies. (2001). *The Nature of the extended/expanded role of nursing.* Retrieved June 24, 2005 from www.cns.nf.ca

Chang, K.P.K., Wong, T. (2001). The nurse specialist role in Hong Kong: Perceptions of nurse specialists. *Journal of Advanced Nursing*, **36**(1), 32–40.

Chao, Y.M.Y. (2005). *Designing nurse practitioner system in Taiwan.* Paper delivered at the 23rd ICN Congress, Taipei.

Chen, C.H. *Nurse practitioner/advanced practice nursing roles in Taiwan.* Education /Practice Subgroup of the International Nurse Practitioner/Advanced Practice Nursing Network. Retrieved June 15, 2005 from http://icn-apnetwork.org/

Cho, H.S.M., Kashka, M.S. (2004). The evolution of the community health nurse practitioner in Korea. *Public Health Nursing*, **21**:3, 287–294.

Danielson, E. (2003). New initiatives and developments in advanced practice and NP roles. Paper given at the ICN Conference Geneva. Retrieved 7 June, 2005 from http://icn-apnetwork.org/

Duffy E. (2002). *Global definition and characteristics of nurse practitioners/advanced practice nurses.* Report of an ICN International Nurse Practitioner/Advanced Practice Nurse Survey. Unpublished.

Fahey-Walsh, J. (2004). *Literature review report. Advanced nursing practice and the primary health care nurse practitioner: Title, scope, and role.* Canadian Nurse Practitioner Initiative. Retrieved 24 June, 2005 from http://www.cnpi.ca/documents/pdf/Practice_Role_Title_Scope_Literature_Review_e.pdf

Gardner, G., Carryer, J., Dunn, S.V., Gardner, A. (2004). *Nurse practitioner standards project.* Queensland University of Technology, Australian Nursing Council.

International Council of Nurses. (2001). *Update: International survey of nurse practitioner/advanced practice nursing roles.* Retrieved June 30, 2005 from http://icn-apnetwork.org/

International Council of Nurses. (2002). *Definition and characteristics of the role.* Retrieved June 21, 2005 from http://www.icn-apnetwork.org

International Council of Nurses Credentialing Forum. (2002). *Japan country report for the Credentialing Forum.* Unpublished.

International Council of Nurses Credentialing Forum. (2004a). *Japan country report.* Unpublished.

International Council of Nurses Credentialing Forum. (2004b). *Jamaica country report.* Unpublished.

International Council of Nurses Credentialing Forum. (2005a). *Denmark country report.* Unpublished.

International Council of Nurses Credentialing Forum. (2005b). *Japan country report.* Unpublished.

International Council of Nurses Credentialing Forum. (2005c). *Spain country report.* Unpublished.

International Federation of Nurse Anaesthetists. (2004). *About the International Federation of Nurse Anaesthetists.* Retrieved 13 October, 2005 from http://www.ifna.info/about.asp

Jamieson, L., Willliams, L.M. (2002). Confusion prevails in defining 'advanced nursing practice'. *Collegian*, **9**(4), 29–33.

JNA News. (2002). *5th Year for CEN & CNR Systems*, 32, March.

Jordanian Nursing Council. (2004). *National strategy on nursing*. Amman: Author. Unpublished.

Keeling, A.W., Bigbee, J.L. (2005). The history of advanced practice nursing in the United States. In A.B. Hamric, J.A. Spross, C.M. Hanson (Eds) *Advanced Practice Nursing: An Integrative Approach*, 3rd Edition, pp. 3–43. St. Louis: Elsevier. Saunders.

Ketefian, S., Redman, R.W., Hanucharurnkul, S., Masterson, A., Neves, E.P. (2001). The development of advanced practice roles: Implications in the international nursing community. *International Nursing Review*, **48**, 152–163.

Kim, D.D. (2003). *The APN in Korea*. Presented at the ICN Conference, Geneva, 2003.

Loke, A.Y., Wong, F.K.Y. (2005). *An initiative in developing nurse practitioners in Hong Kong*. Paper delivered at the 23rd ICN Congress, Taipei.

Lorensen, M., Jones, D.E., Hamilton, G.A. (1998). Advanced practice nursing in the Nordic countries. *Journal of Clinical Nursing*, **7**, 257–264.

Munjanja, O.K., Kibuka, S., Dovlo, D. (2005). The nursing workforce in sub-Saharan Africa. Issue Paper No 7 in *The Global Nursing Review Initiative*, Geneva, International Council of Nurses. Retrieved 26 June, 2005 from http://www.icn.ch/global/

National Nursing Organizations of Australia. (2003). *National consensus statement on nurse practitioners*. Australia: Author. Retrieved July 7, 2005 from http://www.anf.org.au/nno/pdf/Consensus_statement.pdf

New Zealand Ministry of Health. (2002). *Nurse practitioners in New Zealand*. Wellington: Author.

New Zealand Nurses Organization. (2000). *Advanced nursing practice: NZNO position statement*. Wellington: Author.

Nurse Practitioner Association of Ontario. *History*. Retrieved July 5, 2005 from http://www.npao.org/history.aspx

Nursing and Midwifery Council. (2005). *NMC consultation on a proposed framework for the standard for post-registration nursing*. London: Author.

Nursing Council of New Zealand. (2002). *The nurse practitioner: Responding to health needs in New Zealand*. Wellington: Author.

Nursing Council of New Zealand. (2004). *Scopes of practice*. Retrieved June 14, 2005 from http://www.nursingcouncil.org.nz/scopes.html

Pan-American Health Organization-World Health Organization. (1999). *Nursing in the region of the Americas. Organization and Management of Health Systems and Services (HSO)*. Washington: Author.

Radebe, G. (2000). Nursing training for the district health system. *HST Update*, 24.

Roodbol, P. (2004). Survey carried out prior to the 3rd ICN-International Nurse Practitioner/Advanced Nursing Practice Network Conference, Gronigen, The Netherlands.

Royal College of Nursing. (2002, revised 2005). *Nurse practitioner: An RCN guide to the nurse practitioner role, competencies and programme approval*. London: Author.

Schober, M. (2002). *Advanced practice: A global perspective*, Paper given at the 2nd ICN International Nurse Practitioner/Advanced Practice Nursing Network Conference, Adelaide.

Schober, M. (2005). *The education and evaluation of nurse practitioner competence: An international perspective*. Paper given at the 21st Annual Nursing Research Conference, Taipei.

Schober, M., Affara, F.A. (2001). *The family nurse. Frameworks for practice*. [Monograph 9]. Geneva, International Council of Nurses.

Schober, M., McKay, N. (2004). *Collaborative practice in the 21st century*. [Monograph 13] Geneva: International Council of Nurses.

Seitio, O.S. (2000). *The family nurse practitioner in Botswana: Issues and challenges*. Presented at the 8th International Nurse Practitioner Conference, San Diego.

Singapore Ministry of Health. (2005). The Nurses & Midwives (Amendment) Bill. Retrieved 8 July, 2005 from http://www.moh.gov.sg/corp/about/newsroom/speeches/details.do?id=31227981

South African Nursing Council. (2004). *Charter of nursing practice, Draft 1*. Pretoria: Author. Retrieved 1 August, 2005 from http://www.sanc.co.za/newsi401.htm

Styles, M.M., Affara, F.A. (1997). *ICN on regulation: Towards a 21*st *century model*. Geneva: International Council of Nurses.

Turner, C., Keyzer, D. (2002). Nurse practitioners: A contract for change and excellence in nursing. *Collegian*, **9**(4), 18–23.

United Kingdom Central Council. (1999). *A higher level of practice: A report of the consultation of the UKCC's proposal for a revised regulatory framework for post-registration clinical practice*. London: Author.

Victorian Government Department of Human Services. (2000). *The Victorian nurse practitioner project: Final report of the taskforce*. Melbourne: Author.

White, M. (2001). *Nurse practitioner/advanced practice in UK*. Retrieved June 15, 2005 from http://icn-apnetwork.org/

Woods, L.P. (2000). *The enigma of advanced nursing practice*. Salisbury, Wilts: Mark Allen.

World Health Organization. (1985). Nurses lead the way. *WHO Features*, 85.

World Health Organization. (2002). *Human resources, national health systems. Shaping the agenda for action. Final report*. Geneva: Author.

World Health Organization. (2002). *Nursing and midwifery services: Strategic directions 2002–2008*. Geneva: WHO.

World Health Organization-Eastern Mediterranean Region. (2001). *Fifth meeting of the Regional Advisory Panel on Nursing and consultation on advanced practice nursing and nurse prescribing: Implications for regulation, nursing education and practice in the Eastern Mediterranean*. WHO-EM/NUR/348/E/L. Cairo: Author.

World Health Organization-Western Pacific Region. (2001). *Mid-level and nurse practitioners in the Pacific: Models and issues*. Manila: Author.

Chapter 2
Nature of practice

Introduction

The nature of advanced nursing practice reflects the position and progress of professional nursing in health care provision. As discussed in Chapter 1, international and national organisations, ministries of health, professional associations and interested individuals are commenting on and studying the phenomenon of advanced nursing practice. While interest is rapidly increasing, certain questions arise: What is it about advanced nursing practice that differentiates it from what has been associated with traditional practice in the field of nursing? What are the factors that drive practice development?

In exploring the nature of advanced nursing practice, the authors recognise that all nurses perform assessments and act in response to their conclusions. A central characteristic of advanced practice is the extent and depth to which that appraisal is made. This brings with it increased levels of accountability and responsibility in making the decisions based on this advanced assessment (American Academy of Nurse Practitioners [AANP], 2002a; Castledine, 1996; Daly & Carnwell, 2003; Gardner *et al.*, 2004) At a very fundamental level advanced and generalist nursing practice differ in definition, characteristics, scope of practice and education. This chapter aims to explore the nature of advanced nursing practice and strives to describe the aspects of practice that distinguish it from generalist nursing.

In describing the nature of advanced nursing practice the authors have attempted to adhere to the following terminology. Role characteristics are viewed as features or qualities that make the advanced practice role recognisable. Competencies refer to the ability of the advanced practice nurse (APN) to do something well to a defined standard. Criteria are accepted standards used in making decisions or judgements about the level of quality or excellence that are accepted as the norm by which actual achievements are judged (e.g. level of education and credentialing for practice). Performance, as related to core competencies, is viewed as the manner in which the APN functions or behaves when providing services. Scope of practice is described as the range of activities covered by advanced practice, while recognising that a critical issue in defining scope is the context in which the advanced practice roles are introduced and implemented. In reviewing aspects of current literature relating to the nature of advanced nursing practice the authors point out that the terms characteristics and competencies are at times used interchangeably thus adding to the confusion in developing clear conceptual models or frameworks for advanced nursing practice.

In conceptualising advanced nursing practice, the use of models or frameworks can be useful in describing the nature and intent of the role. In reviewing frameworks present in the literature, Spross and Lawson (2005) note that domain of practice and competency can be seen as the most common concepts used in explaining the nature of advanced nursing practice, but the meaning attributed to these concepts is inconsistent. For examples of conceptual frameworks and models developed for this purpose, refer to the Hamric model (Figure 2.1) and the Brown framework (Figure 2.2) as attempts to point out conceptually the nature of advanced nursing practice.

The current Hamric model is based on literature from all APN specialties, but the early conceptual model derived from the CNS role (Hamric, 1996). Revisions and refinement have occurred over time reflecting the changes in practice, increased research and a better understanding of a theoretical basis for advanced nursing practice. Hamric (2005) conceptualises advanced nursing practice:

Advanced practice nursing is the application of an expanded range of practical, theoretical, and research-based competencies to phenomena experienced by patients within a specialised clinical area of the larger discipline of nursing (p. 89).

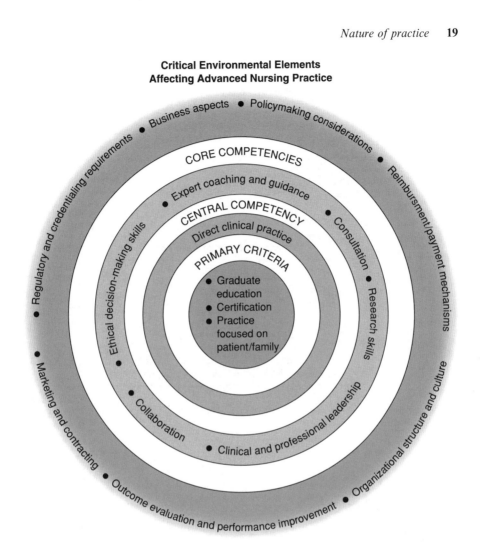

Figure 2.1 Hamric's model for advanced nursing practice. (Source: Hamric, 2005, with permission.)

This model (Figure 2.1) proposes an integrative understanding of the core of advanced nursing practice. The conceptual definition and defining characteristics include:

> *primary criteria (graduate education, certification in the specialty, and a focus on clinical practice with patients) and a set of core competencies (direct clinical practice, collaboration, coaching and guidance, research, ethical decision-making, consultation and leadership).*

Brown (1998) provides a framework that is comprehensive in that it addresses both the nature of practice and the context in which the practice occurs.

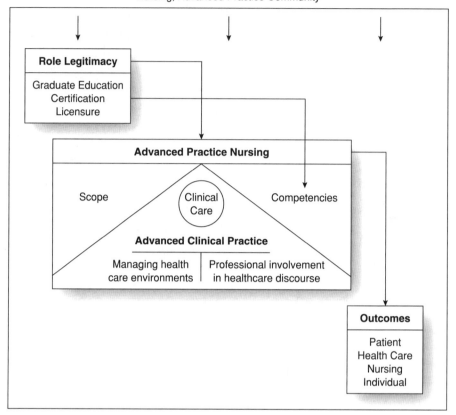

Figure 2.2 Brown's framework for advanced nursing practice. (Source: Brown, 1998, with permission.)

The significance of a nursing orientation is taken into consideration, while at the same time noting that the advanced nursing role includes skills often associated with medical practice. The framework (Figure 2.2) utilises domains and competencies that could be used for the purposes of: 'differentiating practice, designing curricula and evaluating advanced practice' (Spross & Lawson, 2005, p. 64). This conceptual framework includes four main and 17 specific concepts with the central concept being advanced nursing practice. The four main concepts (with the related specific concepts in brackets) are: 'environments (society, health-care economy, local conditions, nursing, advanced practice community); role legitimacy (graduate education, certification, licensure); advanced practice nursing (scope, clinical care, competencies, managing health-care environments, professional involvement in health-care discourse); and outcomes (patient, health-care system, the nursing profession, individual APN outcomes' (Spross & Lawson, 2005, pp. 63–64)).

The Hamric model and the Brown framework both propose an integrative or comprehensive view of advanced nursing practice with direct advanced clinical care at the core. Although the terminology varies, both take into consideration adaptation to environmental factors affecting the growth and development of the APN. The Hamric model provides a set of measurable primary criteria that are core or central elements that must be met before a nurse can be considered an APN. This model originated from a perspective of specialist nursing and has subsequently been adapted for use in broader contexts. Once a generalist nurse has satisfied the primary criteria, the model proposes a move to direct advanced clinical practice as a core competency adding six additional core competencies to clinical practice regardless of role function or setting. The expectation is that at an advanced level of practice advanced competencies are visible and measurable while also noting that direct clinical practice interacts with all additional competencies. This model depicts a potential flow from specialisation to more inclusive practice competencies. The core attributes are surrounded by and affected by contextual and environment factors (Hamric, 2005). The Brown framework also places clinical care as a core component for the APN but within a framework that moves the generalist nurse in a defined direction from establishing role legitimacy to an overarching balance of scope and competencies leading to direct clinical care and resulting in outcomes affecting patients, health care, the nursing profession and the individual. Whereas environmental elements appear to surround and constantly affect the central components of the Hamric model, in the Brown framework role legitimacy, advanced clinical nursing practice and subsequent outcomes appear to be derived from the environmental factors.

These two examples are provided by the authors to promote debate and discussion while also recognising that additional literature and organisational models are available for the reader to consider. Consult the resources section of this book to access additional information on concepts and ideas to utilise in development of a usable framework. Also note that ICN is in the process of developing a framework for APN practice for use as a guideline when looking at the emerging nature of advanced nursing practice.

In discussion on the nature of advanced practice as well as the provision of models and frameworks being used by countries introducing APN roles, the authors recognise the dominance of published literature originating from the United States, Canada and the United Kingdom. In recent years, this has been supplemented by a noticeable increase of published contributions from Australia and New Zealand. Perspectives of advanced nursing practice contributed by key informants and from other published and unpublished sources have enabled the authors to present a broader view of the developments in this field. The expansion and increasing presence of APNs internationally will add to the experiential information as well as provide an impetus for a wider range of research into what constitutes advanced nursing practice. Refer to Chapter 6 for discussion of a research agenda that will assist with this task.

Advanced practice nurse (APN) characteristics

Making a clear distinction between characteristics of advanced versus generalist nursing practice as new roles develop is a demanding but necessary undertaking. It is likely that nurses in other roles may be providing nursing services containing elements of practice similar to those described and identified for advanced practice. In assessing the situation in Australia and New Zealand, Gardner *et al.* (2004) suggest that, as the scope of practice and core competencies of the APN are defined and agreed to over time, it is likely that the ambiguity in the boundaries between advanced practice and other areas of nursing will clarify. This makes it all the more essential that from the initial phase of development and analysis, characteristics expected to be associated with new roles are well articulated and defined.

In describing characteristics of advanced nursing practice, the question presents as to what benchmark determines definition of roles. Schober (2004a) emphasises

> *What characterizes advanced nursing practice is knowledge and expertise, clinical judgement, skilled and self-initiated care, and scholarly inquiry, but not job descriptions, title or setting (p. 3).*

Increasingly leaders, writers, researchers and spokespersons for advanced nursing practice emphasise that, while the principles of practice are firmly rooted in the core of nursing, there is overlap and integration of skills that have historically been attributed to other professions (Castledine, 2003; Coleman & Fox, 2003; Gardner *et al.*, 2004; Roberts-Davis & Read, 2002; key informants, personal communication).

Adopting phrases such as 'physician substitutes' or 'mini-doctors' or 'physician extenders' tends to focus only on those characteristics that appear similar to, or are traits associated with, medical practice. There is a tendency in the literature to continually compare APN and physician practice, thus setting up an adversarial relationship. Turris *et al.* (2005) in an editorial rebuttal note that 'the value is not in the role functions that overlap, as in the role functions that are unique' (p. 2). The authors of this book propose that it is the merging of nursing values and expertise with advanced knowledge, clinical judgement and decision-making skills in providing a nursing service that forms the essence of advanced practice, and contributes an additional dimension to provision of health care services.

ICN official position on APN characteristics

To facilitate common understanding, as well as to guide further international development, ICN (2002) has identified the characteristics of the advanced practice nurse. The characteristics reflect current roles and the potential for development of advanced nursing practice worldwide. These characteristics as given in Figure 2.3 are to be seen as guidelines to aim for in the process of role

Educational Preparation

- Educational preparation at an advanced level
- Formal recognition of educational programmes
- A formal system of licensure, registration, certification or credentialing

Nature of Practice

- The ability to integrate research, education and clinical management
- High degree of autonomy and independent practice
- Case management
- Advanced assessment and decision-making skills
- Recognized advanced clinical competencies
- The ability to provide consultant services to other health professionals
- Recognized first point of entry for services

Regulatory Mechanism – country specific regulations that underpin APN practice

- Right to diagnose
- Authority to prescribe medications and treatments
- Authority to refer to other professionals
- Authority to admit to hospital
- Title protection
- Legislation specific to advanced practice

Figure 2.3 ICN characteristic for the advanced practice nurse. (Source: ICN, 2002.)

development, and do not necessarily represent the current status in all countries where advanced practice nurses are present.

Country illustrations

Country illustrations are presented in order to portray actual examples of advanced nursing role characteristics.

In Botswana solidifying nursing's contribution to health care services was essential. Initially emphasis was placed on assessment, diagnosis and management of common diseases, in addition to health promotion and disease prevention. Nurses developed advanced clinical skills through undertaking further education which integrated theory from nursing, social, medical and public health (key informant, personal communication).

Following definition of the nature of practice and role characteristics, NPs in the United States have carved out a distinctive presence over a forty year period by establishing title recognition, regulatory authority, educational and credentialing standards (Towers, 2005; key informants, personal communication). This did not happen rapidly and occurred as other advanced roles of the clinical nurse specialist (CNS), nurse midwife (NMW) and nurse anaesthetist (NA) were also evolving (Keeling & Bigbee, 2005).

In the Cayman Islands the initiation of comprehensive health care services started in 1930 with provision of care by a local midwife when physicians were scarce and conditions were primitive. Primary health care progressed with the official employment of a nurse in 1990 who was able to diagnose, treat, prescribe and dispense what was viewed to be necessary for whatever cases present in the island settings. There was backup consultation by phone to the nearest hospital, or by appointment for the periodic visiting physician clinics. The multi-faceted role includes counsellor, administrator, staff supervisor, health educator, accountant and secretary in addition to advanced clinical assessment and management skills (Schober, 2004b).

The Canadian Nurses Association's (CNA, 2002) national framework for advanced nursing practice recommends characteristics that are associated with a broad definition consistent with expert and specialised practice. The terms 'expanded' and 'extended' are used to describe practice characteristics including competencies that are considered to be outside the scope of nursing practice. The roles of CNS and NP are similar in many ways, but the roles also have unique characteristics. Most noteworthy of these is that while NPs have prescriptive and diagnostic authority, this does not apply to the CNS. Differences in characteristics extend beyond role titles in that individuals with the same title can carry out the role differently depending on educational preparation, scope of practice, area of specialisation, organisational structure, province/territory of residence, and provincial regulatory and health care legislation (key informants, personal communication).

Community health nurse practitioners (CHNP) in South Korea provide health education, disease management, immunisations, school health services and care for the elderly in agrarian communities. Characteristics of the role that has been in existence for over 20 years include performing physical examinations, screening or clinic consultations, diagnosis, prescriptive authority and referral to other practitioners. In addition, the CHNP provides home visits, lectures to the community on health topics, as well as after-hour phone calls for acute and urgent problems (Schober, 2004b).

In Switzerland new advanced practice hospital-based roles include many of the ICN (2002) recommended characteristics. However, education in the skill of using scientific literature as well as the ability to evaluate and argue ethical questions effectively has been given special emphasis. The Swiss focus has been to deepen understanding in clinical sciences relevant to practice (key informant, personal communication).

Hong Kong, Singapore, Taiwan and Japan describe characteristics that are congruent with those described in the ICN official position, but differ most often in aspects related to the degree of autonomy ascribed to the role, the ability to prescribe or diagnose, as well as the availability of the APN to be first point of contact for services (key informants, personal communication).

Labelling the role

Titling

A clearly identifiable title that indicates levels of responsibility, accountability and performance central to the role is helpful in the debate and discussion surrounding the nature of practice. However, it is worth noting that for the authors to attempt to establish a clear description of the nature of advanced practice from this perspective alone is an undertaking fraught with difficulty. Functions and responsibility vary considerably from one setting to another in relationship to commonly used titles such as 'nurse practitioner', 'advanced practice nurse', 'advanced nursing practice', 'nurse specialist' and 'clinical nurse specialist' even in the same country.

The diversity in use of titles appears to originate not only from varying forces that have influenced role development in a specific country, but also from the familiarity of key stakeholders with countries where there is a longer history of advanced nursing roles. A number of nations have introduced or developed a title based on service needs, as in Botswana, South Korea and the Netherlands. Educational institutions have introduced APN or NP titles while planning new masters level nursing education programmes in the absence of role definition. For example, at Aga Khan University School of Nursing in Karachi, in Pakistan and at Hong Kong Polytechnic University School of Nursing the educational perspective and educational experiences of faculty rather than the needed role have determined titling for advanced practice. In the absence of definitive standards and legal parameters, title variance is found in states, provinces and institutions within the same region, country or locale, as in Australia, Canada, the United Kingdom, the United States (key informants, personal communication), as well as islands in the Pacific (World Health Organization-Western Pacific Region [WHO-WPRO], 2001).

The authors could find no clearly identifiable processes specific to skills, knowledge acquisition or special competencies of advanced nursing practice that are obviously associated with title selection. It appears that the diversity in titles reflects the random nature of the process used when titles are originally selected (Castledine, 2003; Gardner *et al.*, 2004). Advanced nursing practice or advanced practice nursing tend to be used as umbrella terms embracing more specific titles that are associated with advanced nursing roles such as nurse practitioner, clinical nurse specialist, nurse midwife, nurse anaesthetist, as in the United States (Hanson, 2005; Towers, 2005; key informants, personal communication) or primary health care nurse practitioner and clinical nurse specialist as in Canada (CNA, 2002; key informants, personal communication).

Throughout this book the authors have used advanced nursing practice to take full account of this field and to be inclusive in recognising all aspects of clinical nursing considered to be advanced or advancing. The term 'advanced practice nurse' (APN) is used to refer to the specific individual who adopts the role identified as advanced nursing practice.

The use of the title NP could mean a nurse with a master's degree capable of providing generalised comprehensive services in primary health care (PHC) as in Australia, Botswana, Canada, and the United States, or it could signify providing specialised practice in hospital settings as in Iceland, the Netherlands, South Korea, Hong Kong, Singapore and Taiwan (key informants, personal communication). On the other hand, nurse specialists (NS) or CNS are often described as focusing on one specialty such as oncology or cardiology (Castledine, 2002; Cattini & Knowles, 1999; Chan, 2001; Heitkemper, 2004), but at times these responsibilities are similar to what is often associated with a comprehensive NP role. It is not always clear what these distinctions are, and the terms 'advanced', 'specialist' and 'practitioner' are frequently used interchangeably in publications and documents. Lack of formal registration or regulation in many countries adds to the confusion and makes it difficult to compare roles, levels of education and competency across countries (Buchan & Calman, 2004b).

Differences in titling and changing roles worldwide emphasise the necessity to define scope of practice and characteristics describing anticipated functions and services to be provided by the nurse in an advanced role. While a case can be made that it is not the title, but definition of the role itself that is essential (Roberts-Davis & Read, 2001), nevertheless a title remains important as it is the quickest way to communicate who is this health provider. Table 2.1 lists examples of titles used internationally.

Title protection

A title indicates a certain level of expectation with respect to accountability and professional service that this health provider can offer. In the absence of formal title protection, potentially any nurse can assume a title associated with advanced nursing practice without having to demonstrate equivalent competence or undertaking the education required for that level of practice. Chapter 4 contains more discussion on the purpose of title protection and related regulatory issues.

Scope of practice

What is scope of practice?

Scope of practice describes the range of activities associated with recognised professional responsibilities that are in keeping with the limitations imposed by regulatory provisions in the setting where practice occurs. Specifically, the scope describes what an APN can do, what population can be seen or treated, and under what circumstance or guidance the APN can provide care (Hanson, 2005; Klein, 2005). Ethical and cultural conduct, educational requirements, along with aspects of accountability and responsibility for professional actions, form components of scope of practice.

Definitions of scope of practice tend to be broad, allowing for flexibility to respond to a dynamic health care environment and to promote inclusion of the variety of roles that might be present in a country or locale (American Nurses Association [ANA], 1996; AANP, 2002a; 2002b; ICN, 2005). Finally the scope of practice not only provides a description of the accountability and responsibility expected of the APN, but also forms the foundation for developing appropriate and sound educational programmes.

Table 2.1 Advanced practice nurse titles. (Source: Key Informants, personal communication; WHO–WPRO, 2001.)

Country or Region	Title(s) Used
Australia	Nurse Practitioner**
Bahrain	Specialist Nurse*
Botswana	Family Nurse Practitioner*
Canada	Clinical Nurse Specialist, Advanced Practice Nurse, Nurse Practitioner. Acute Care Nurse Practitioner, Specialty Nurse Practitioner, Primary Healthcare Nurse Practitioner, Clinical Nurse Specialist/Nurse Practitioner * & **
France	Nursing approach to a specialty e.g. anaesthesia*
Hong Kong	Advanced Practice Nurse, Nurse Practitioner, Nurse Specialist*
Iceland	Nurse Specialist
Ireland	Advanced Nurse Practitioner (Area of Practice in brackets)
Japan	Certified Nurse Specialist
Jordan	Nurse Specialist
Korea	Advanced Practice Nurse
Macao	Specialist Nurse*
Netherlands	Nursing Specialist (Dutch: Verpleegkundig specialist)
New Zealand	Nurse Practitioner
Philippines	Clinical Nurse Specialist*
Thailand	Clinical Nurse Specialist, Nurse Practitioner
Taiwan	Advanced Practice Nurse* (Official title used in Chinese only)
Singapore	Advanced Practice Nurse*
Sweden	Advanced Nurse Practitioner in Primary Health Care, Advanced Specialist Nurse*
Switzerland	Advanced Practice Nurse, Clinical Nurse Specialist, Nurse Specialist
Republic of South Africa	Advanced Practice Nurse*
UK	Nurse Practitioner, Advanced Nurse, Specialist, Nurse Consultant, Community Matron*
USA	Nurse Practitioner, Clinical Nurse Specialist, Nurse Midwife, Nurse Anaesthetist, Advanced Practice Registered Nurse**
Western Pacific	Nurse Practitioner or Mid-level Practitioner * & **

* Official Title Recognition pending
** Varies among the states, provinces or islands

For those countries with new advanced practice initiatives, the scope of practice may initially arise from practice acts and standards that are normally associated with the generalist nurse. At times this is helpful because these regulations and standards for nursing provide a foundation for role development. For advanced nursing practice, the problem arises when there is a reluctance to move beyond the generalist nurse focus to develop standards that will underpin the more complex knowledge and skill sets that APNs bring to practice. Support, openness, fresh ideas and a willingness to take risks by nursing and other professional bodies, as well as governmental organisations, is most crucial in activating and sustaining a new scope of practice if nursing is to advance.

Dunning (2002) recommends that the advanced nursing practice definition describe a general scope of practice appropriate to national and professional needs. In settings with highly specialised APN roles, a specific scope of practice can be developed, while making sure that it is built on and is consistent with the intents of the generic advanced practice scope. The New Zealand experience illustrates this perspective in that the specialty areas are organised under a generic scope, while NPs delineate their own specialty or subspecialty scope of practice (Nursing Council New Zealand [NCNZ], 2002).

What influences development of scope of practice?

A joint statement by Canadian nurses, pharmacists and physicians notes that the primary purpose of defining scopes of practice 'is to meet the health care needs . . . and to serve the interests of patients and the public safely, efficiently, and competently' (Canadian Medical Association *et al.*, 2003). While certain general principles apply across all professional scopes of practice, factors such as: fluctuations in, and the composition of, the health care workforce; geographic and economic disparities in access to health care services; economic incentives for health care providers; and consumer demand and the level of understanding of advanced practice roles can influence the final definition. Promoting a flexible, expansive scope of practice for the APN will probably be more difficult in a setting where there is high competition among health professionals than in situations where there is an urgent need for a versatile workforce and integration of skills (Buchan & Calman, 2004b).

In referring to the 1994 United Kingdom Central Council (UKCC) definition of advanced practice as a distinct 'sphere of nursing', Castledine (2003, p. 10) promotes development of scope of practice in the generalist field rather than through specialist practice. This view led the author to propose seven categories as key criteria that could provide a foundation for development of the advanced nursing scope of practice. These categories of key criteria are autonomous practitioner; experienced and knowledgeable, researcher and evaluator of care; expert in health and nursing assessment; expert in case management; consultant; educator and leader; and role model. The criteria emphasise that core nursing principles should guide *advanced clinical nursing practice* (p. 11). Castledine's advice from the United Kingdom perspective is consistent with the recommendations from Dunning's (2002) Australian experience, New Zealand documents (Ministry of Health New Zealand 2002; NCNZ, 2002) as well as a study conducted in the United Kingdom by Roberts-Davis and Read (2001).

When comparing models or scope of practice statements in the Western Pacific (World Health Organization-Western Pacific Region [WHO-WPRO], 2001) it is noted that there is no one best fit to identify the dimensions of advanced nursing practice, as in these circumstances practice is dictated by what is best for the country's particular situation. In this region a wide range of curative and preventive services is provided within what appears to be a broad, flexible and somewhat vague scope of practice. In Thailand where there is as yet no published scope of practice, advanced nursing activities are delineated by a Thai Nursing Council protocol (key informants, personal communication).

Points to consider when defining scope of practice

As previously discussed, scope of practice statements should promote safe, ethical practice and the delivery of quality health care services. Scope statements should distinguish between the different categories of nursing personnel, and make clear the distinctive practice of the category of nurse practising under the scope.

Usually a scope of practice communicates:

- The body of knowledge, values, attitudes and skills (indicating required level and depth judgement, critical thinking, analysis, problem solving, decision making, leadership) of the health care provider
- The roles expected of the health care provider (e.g. direct care giver, case manager, educator, advocate, researcher, planner and evaluator of health services)
- The nature of the client population in terms of complexity of health problems to be the focus of care, and the comprehensiveness of the services required
- The degree of accountability, responsibility and authority that the health care provider assumes for the outcome of his or her practice.

When setting out to define the scope of advanced nursing practice, it is critical to remember that it grows out of the scope defined for the generalist nurse. The generalist nurse scope is the starting point, and the task will be to define how the scope of advanced nursing practice expands beyond that of the generalist nurse in terms of roles, functions, types of client populations and accountability. The questions that follow can help in checking progress during this process.

- Does it fit with the definitions and values that underpin nursing?
- Does the scope contribute to meeting public need and demand for APN services?
- Is it sufficiently complex and advanced so that it is clearly beyond the scope of general nursing practice, requiring advanced and more in-depth education?

- Is the scope based on a core body of nursing knowledge that is being continually expanded and refined by research?
- Are there the legalisation, regulations, policies guidelines to support the expanded roles and function? If not what will have to be done to ensure that the APN is working within a legal scope of practice e.g. legislative change, adoption of policies/guidelines/protocols to support APN practice within the scope defined?

ICN, consistent with its mandate to provide global leadership in the field of nursing practice, is consulting with its international networks and others on a scope of practice for use by countries seeking to develop or refine their own scopes. The scope being developed is intended to facilitate understanding and stimulate discussion as to what would be appropriate for a given context. The ICN scope will propose areas of knowledge and technical abilities necessary for the qualified APN to practice safely, ethically and with cultural sensitivity when performing acts, procedures, and implementing protocols and practice guidelines. It will make the point that the clinical practice of the APN is scientifically based and applicable to health care practice in primary, secondary and tertiary settings, in urban and rural communities. The scope will take account of the APN role in the areas of patient and peer education, mentorship, leadership and management, including the responsibility to translate, utilise and undertake meaningful research to advance and improve nursing practice. Examples of scopes of practice from several countries are given in Appendix 2.

Core competencies

Core competencies or performance competencies are commonly used in describing APN roles (Cattini & Knowles, 1999; Maclaine *et al.*, 2004; National Organization of Nurse Practitioner Faculties [NONPF], 2000; 2002; RCN, 2002) but the concept of assigning or determining role competencies is controversial. Competence is defined in a variety of ways. In an extensive literature review of clinical competence Watson *et al.* (2002) found that there appeared to be universal acceptance of the need to assess clinical nursing competence, but published literature did not demonstrate the reliability and validity of this approach. Girot (2000) further pointed out the problematic issue of differentiating different levels of competence. Competency-based practice within the context of advanced nursing may unreasonably restrict role development while failing to recognise that nursing principles and values form the foundation of advanced practice (McAllister, 1998). Regardless of the inconsistencies and controversies surrounding the use of role competencies, the notion of applying this concept occupies the attention of regulatory authorities as it is seen to be a way to demonstrate safe APN practice. Without a better alternative, competence, competencies and core competencies will probably continue to be used as a way to measure or standardise advanced nursing practice.

In summarising data from research findings collected in Australia and New Zealand and after an extensive literature review Gardner *et al.* (2004) determined that the core role of the nurse practitioner is characterised by autonomous extended practice requiring advanced clinical knowledge and skills in stable, variable and complicated conditions. Findings by these researchers underline a concept of *competency and capability* (p. 2) as essential components for NP practice. The Canadian Nurses Association (CNA, 2002) identifies advanced nursing practice core competencies as clinical practice, research, leadership, collaboration and change agent. The CNA framework (2002) describes an identified set of core competencies fundamentally linked to role characteristics. In Ireland (National Council for the Professional Development of Nursing and Midwifery, 2001; 2004), core competencies are linked to a specific post, and emerge from the job analysis process undertaken prior to approving an advanced practice post.

In order to be identified as an NP in New Zealand, an individual must meet the assessment criteria and competencies specified by the Nursing Council (NCNZ, 2002). In analysing and discussing the possibility of advanced practice in the Philippines (Professional Regulation Commission, Board of Nursing, Manila, 2002) key stakeholders determined that 'competence' and 'dimensions of competence performance' are derived from del Bueno's concept of competency assessment and evaluation. The work done by del Bueno and associates challenged hospital-based nurse administrators and managers to implement competency-based practice models such as their Performance-Based Development system (Anthony & del Bueno, 1993; del Bueno, 1995a; 1995b). Having established this core concept, basic competencies in the Philippines are then linked to specialty areas.

Consistent with its practice of identifying core competencies for nursing practice (ICN, 2003a; 2003b) is also developing competencies for the APN. The competencies will arise from the three pillars that ICN believes advances nursing and health care, namely the standards for regulation, practice and socioeconomic welfare. APN competencies proposed by ICN assist with advanced nursing practice development during the formative phase. They are based on the assumptions that:

- Advanced nursing practice is built on the preparation and experience of the generalist nurse.
- Factors in the social, political and economic settings will have an impact on the way the core role and related competencies evolve.

Competencies will support advanced clinical practice taking place within a regulatory framework and an established code of ethics. Implicit in all settings is the view that the APN works in collaboration with other health care professionals.

Listed below are practice competencies already identified and posted on the ICN International NP/APN Network web site for information and feedback. Competencies for professional development are given in Chapter 5 on education.

The APN:

(1)   Uses advanced comprehensive assessment, diagnostic, treatment planning, implementation and evaluation skills

(2)   Applies and adapts advanced skills in complex and/or unstable environments

(3)   Applies sound advanced clinical reasoning and decision making to inform, guide and teach in practice

(4)   Documents assessment, diagnosis, management and monitors treatment and follow-up care in partnership with the patient

(5)   Prescribes and dispenses treatments according to the authorised scope of practice, guidelines and/or protocols

(6)   Uses applicable communication, counselling, advocacy and interpersonal skills to initiate, develop and discontinue therapeutic relationships

(7)   Refers to and accepts referrals from other health care professionals to maintain continuity of care

(8)   Practises independently where authorised and the regulatory framework allows in the interest of the patients, families and communities

(9)   Consults with and is consulted by other health care professionals and others

(10) Works in collaboration with health team members in the interest of the patient

(11) Develops a practice that is based on current scientific evidence and incorporated into the health management of patients, families and communities

(12) Introduces, tests, evaluates and manages evidence based practice

(13) Uses research to produce evidence based practice to improve the safety, efficiency and effectiveness of care

(14) Engages in ethical practice in all aspects of the APN role responsibility

(15) Accepts accountability and responsibility for own advanced professional, judgement, actions, and continued competence

(16) Creates and maintains a safe therapeutic environment through the use of risk management strategies and quality improvement

(17) Assumes leadership and management responsibilities in the delivery of efficient advanced practice nursing services in a changing health care system

(18) Acts as an advocate for patients in the health care systems and the development of health policies that promote and protect the individual patient, family and community

(19) Adapts practice to the contextual and cultural milieu. (ICN, 2005)

Competency: the basis for education and practice

Competency-based education has emerged as a favoured approach to assessing professional performance and delivering professional education (Guilbert, 1987; Jamieson, 1993; Lenburg, 1999a; Uys, 2004). In competency-based education clearly specified outcomes of learning are identified at the early stage of course-planning. Statements of competence and attainment define what students are expected to learn. Competence is defined as 'the effective application of a combination of knowledge, skill and judgement demonstrated by an individual in daily practice or job performance' (ICN, 1997, updated 2004). In nursing, competence reflects the following:

- Knowledge, understanding and judgement
- Skills: cognitive, technical or psychomotor and interpersonal
- A range of personal attributes and attitudes (ICN, 1997).

One of the useful educational models based on competencies is Lenburg's (1999b) **C**ompetency **O**utcome **P**erformance **A**ssessment model (COPA). This requires the integration of practice-based outcomes with interactive learning and performance assessment of competencies delivered within an educational environment that values interactive student-focused learning. It requires faculty to examine four basic questions during the process of curriculum development:

- What are the essential competencies and outcomes for contemporary practice?
- What are the indicators that define those competencies?
- What are the most effective ways to learn those competencies, and
- What are the most effective ways to document that learners and/or practitioners have achieved the required competencies? (Lenburg, 1999b)

Lenburg's (1999b) eight core practice competencies dealing with assessment and intervention; communication; critical thinking; teaching; human caring relationships; management; leadership; and knowledge integration skills form the basis of a practice-based profession. Applying the **COPA** model when identifying APN competencies is useful because of its focus on practice. The eight core areas form a constellation around which sets of competencies can be identified for APN practice.

Creating a competency map

To develop a curriculum around professional competencies, a process is needed to identify competencies and create a competency map which provides a profile or role definition of advanced nursing practice. The COPA model has been suggested as a useful approach to this task. As competencies cannot be identified from an 'armchair', a method capable of delineating those required for the APN to fulfil the role-related responsibilities recognised in the scope of practice are needed. Usually a combination of several approaches is used in the process:

- Situational analysis which builds up a clearer picture of the context in which the competencies are to be demonstrated.
- Functional analysis which seeks to identify the key purposes and roles of advanced nursing practice.

- Scope of practice definitions.
- Observation of the expert practitioner which is a useful way to obtain information about the APN-patient/client interaction.
- Creating representative scenarios describing situations likely to be met by the advanced nurse practitioners followed by analysis for specific knowledge, skills, judgement and attitude requirements.
- Analysis of critical incidents which serves to identify the attributes regarded as essential to competent, successful practice (Ballantyne *et al.*, 1998; Perry, 1997). An incident is an example of particularly effective or ineffective practice. It leads to a behaviour or response where it is possible to infer the consequences of the behaviour displayed by the practitioner. Also the use of *critical* implies that the behaviour has a significant positive or negative impact on the outcome. To use this technique there needs to be a set of procedures for systematically documenting (e.g. through observations, interviews and self-reports) what actually happened *before, during, and after* which contributed to the successful or failed behaviour. By collecting a sufficient number of such critical incidents it is possible to build a profile of the competencies that are required for satisfactory performance in any professional group.
- Use of expert practitioners to speak about what they do. Asking them to define their role and make more explicit what knowledge, skills and judgements they need in their practice enables a deeper exploration of those areas that are not explicitly observable.
- Literature reviews.
- Expert review of suggested competencies.

When countries are at the very beginning of developing the advanced practice role, access to expert practitioners may be minimal, and there will be greater reliance on competencies already identified by international and/or national groups. Assistance from outside expert practitioners is helpful in guiding this task. However, as a country develops its APN cadre it can begin to draw on their experience, and, through a process of ongoing review, competencies should begin to better reflect the particular focus and health needs of its population.

Formulating competency statements

A competency statement focuses on the outcome of the performance or learning experience. The most important element to remember is that competency statements should refer to the performance of the practitioner. In education the term 'learning outcome' is used to indicate the competence to be achieved at the end of the teaching-learning experience. It is important to use clear and unambiguous language which encourages a uniform interpretation. One of the major challenges is to identify behaviours (actions) at the higher end of the cognitive (mental skills), affective (feelings and emotions) and psychomotor manual or physical skills) domains (Bloom, 1956; Bloom *et al.*, 1965) as that will be the level of practice expected of the APN. Competencies and skills requiring a lower level of functioning may be subsumed under each of the higher level competencies.

According to Uys (2004), four components are usually present in a *full* competency statement. It consists of:

(1) A title which identifies the competency and distinguishes it from others. It should be clear, unique and descriptive, e.g. **Physical assessment of adult.**

(2) Begins with the element of competence (cognitive, psychomotor, affective, relational) which stipulates what a person should be able to do or exhibit, e.g. **Conducts a systematic and comprehensive physical assessment.**

(3) Performance criteria which stipulate how well something should be done. Performance criteria should be achievable and measurable and relate directly to the competency, e.g. **Communicates in a culturally sensitive manner; adjusts the examination to the age, sex, physical and mental condition; obtains accurate data; orders appropriate laboratory tests; records findings systematically, accurately and clearly.**

(4) Range statements describing the conditions, circumstances and/or settings under which the competency should be demonstrated, e.g. **In clinical (inpatient, outpatient) and community-based (e.g. home, workplace) settings.**

The reader is encouraged to consult *Competency in Nursing* (Uys, 1994) for a detailed step by step approach to using competencies in practice, education and regulation. The work of Bloom and his colleagues are a source of useful verbs to describe higher order levels of thinking, feeling and doing (Bloom, 1956; Bloom *et al.*, 1965).

Advanced tasks versus advanced nursing roles

Tasks do not define a profession; the professional viewpoint of practice guides the principles and nature of the related activities (Carryer, 2002). Nurses who have taken on tasks or expertise traditionally associated with medicine suggest that adopting these tasks is a 'means of increasing access and improving services rather than a change in the philosophical approach to practice' (Gardner *et al.*, 2004, p. 47). New and advanced tasks are viewed as valid components of advanced nursing when they provide a convenience for patients and families and offer an opportunity to enhance quality, comprehensiveness and continuity of health care services.

The authority to carry out advanced technical skills and tasks, although beneficial to health care provision, should not be considered as the fundamental distinguishing feature separating advanced nursing practice from generalist nursing. Advanced level tasks are components of the full scope but do not define the essence of advanced practice. In the early years of advanced nursing practice development in the United Kingdom, Bowling and Stilwell (1988) pointed out that while skills and tasks are integral to the APN role, the core values and foundations of advanced practice are derived from a 'philosophy of auto-nomous nursing practice and accountability for that practice' (p. 29). The ability to develop a perspective beyond tasks is that factor that promotes APN roles that are nursing-centred as well advanced in nature.

Controversial practice topics

Differences in the starting points in the growth of advanced nursing practice and subsequent development are of interest as they demonstrate the way specific factors influence advancement. Whereas in certain settings dealing with practice topics such as prescribing, diagnosing and the granting of hospital privileges is avoided because it raises real or perceived areas of disagreement; in other situations these same components are addressed from the beginning. This section discusses these three controversial aspects of advanced practice, and suggests some questions to be explored when considering whether to include these components in the scope of practice for advanced nurses.

Prescriptive authority

> Should all APNs have the right to prescribe medications and other therapeutic agents?
>
> Is prescriptive authority an option or a necessity for advanced practice?
>
> How restrictive should the regulations be for APN prescribing?
>
> Will advanced nursing practice progress without the authority to prescribe or dispense medicines?
>
> What guidelines, protocols or formularies assure competence while protecting the public?

In appraising the international situation with respect to nurse prescribing, Buchan & Calman (2004a) indicate that there is 'little consistency across the countries as to exactly what role nurses should take in prescribing' (p. 35). Educational programmes preparing nurses to prescribe range from masters degree study to distance learning or a designated programme of study days. While methods of educational preparation are varied, common approaches for deciding on what model of nurse prescribing is adopted include: the level of acceptance for nurse prescribing within the health care setting; the method for designating which nurses will prescribe; strategies for implementation and the feasibility from an administrative as well as a health policy perspective.

Debate commonly focuses on the suitability of these functions for nurses. Dialogue on this point often reveals that nurses have been prescribing medicines, treatments and other therapies but too often this occurs outside a legal framework. The availability of proper support and legal authority may lag behind the reality of practice. It is worth noting that there is increasing acceptance that for quality PHC services in various areas of the world, prescribing from a specified list of essential drugs is an important part of the nurse's role (WHO, 2001a; 2001b). If advancement in nursing is to take place, prescriptive authority seems to be a requisite.

The concept of prescribing for APNs and nurses in general is a contentious issue that produces a good deal of conflict and anxiety. Other health professionals take issue with the notion that prescribing should ever be included in the domain of nursing. It is important, however, to recognise that prescriptive authority is only one aspect of comprehensive medication management.

Buchan and Calman (2004a) identify four models that describe and discuss how prescribing can be relevant to nursing practice (see Figure 2.4). The proposed models range from autonomous nurse prescribing to a very limited authority for medicine administration under medical supervision. Nurse prescribing is not always associated with advanced practice roles, as in Sweden; but those countries that have successfully implemented nurse prescribing appear to have either well-established community nursing and/or advanced nursing practice roles.

In the United Kingdom, although NPs have an established presence in provision of health care, they do not have prescriptive authority incorporated into their scope of practice. Community or practice nurses already have the authority to prescribe from a limited formulary in their scope, while NPs need to undertake additional educational courses to be able to prescribe (key informants, personal communication). Similarly in Canada prescriptive authority differs among the range of nurses that fall within the advanced practice category. While the NP has prescriptive authority, the CNS does not have this option (key informants, personal communication). New Zealand, from the beginning of NP development, has supported the right of the NP to prescribe if the appropriate education is acquired and approval given (MOHNZ, 2002). This was strengthened with the identification of what additional qualifications are required for NPs seeking registration with prescribing rights (New Zealand Gazette, 2002). In September 2005, after several years of negotiation, the New Zealand Government extended prescribing rights for nurse practitioners. The list finally approved includes 1379 medications plus a further list of controlled drugs (M. Clark, personal communication).

In a survey looking at trends in NP practice in the United States, data indicate that over 96% of NPs now have some level of prescriptive authority and over 64% of NPs surveyed were authorised to prescribe controlled substances (Goolsby *et al.*, 2005). The American Academy of Nurse Practitioners advocates unlimited prescriptive authority and dispensing privileges within the NP's scope of practice (AANP, 2002b; 2002c). The widespread establishment of prescribing authority in the United States is a result of the gradual introduction

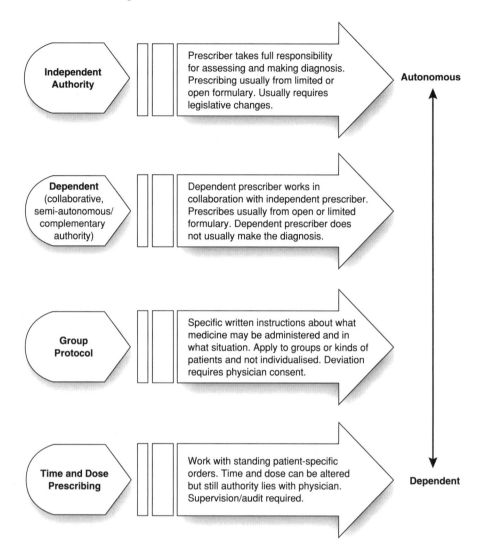

Figure 2.4   Models of nurse prescribing. (Source: Buchan & Calman, 2004b.)

of prescriptive authority and the acceptance that APNs are competent to prescribe safely.

In contrast, in the Republic of Yemen the law prohibits health professionals other than physicians from prescribing even though in practice nurses
and other professionals do prescribe when no doctor is present. Similarly
Sudan provides an example of the lag between legal authority and the reality of
nurse prescribing. Although regulatory support for prescriptive authority does
not exist in the country, nurses providing front-line services are competently prescribing drugs (WHO-EMRO, 2001). In Botswana the regulatory authority is silent
on the issue of nurse prescribing. Although NPs have prescriptive powers, the

limitations of these powers surface when a health facility manager lacks under-standing of the NP role (Seitio, 2000; key informant, personal communication). Midwives in the Republic of South Africa are the one group able to prescribe or dispense drugs. While nurses in advanced roles in the public sector prescribe, authority is limited to the special circumstance created by the absence of medical personnel (key informant, personal communication).

Approaching APN prescribing

Questions to consider in approaching the decision of inclusion of nurse prescribing in the development of APN scope of practice include:

(1) Is there a practice protocol or guideline in the country, locale or facility for nurse prescribing?
(2) Who is responsible for developing protocols and guidelines?
(3) Is there language in any of the professional practice acts or other acts governing management of drugs that prohibit nurse prescribing?
(4) Is there a standard of care reference guidebook that is adhered to by all professionals that influences medication management?
(5) Are there drug formularies for the setting, agency or health care facility that must be adhered to?
(6) What professional or regulatory bodies oversee prescribing, dispensing and drug management in the country?
(7) Does the country use the WHO essential drug formulary?
(8) Will lack of prescriptive authority impact or limit the kind and quality of services provided by the APN?

The diagnosis debate

> Should nurses have the capacity to provide initial diagnosis or a differential diagnosis?
>
> Does differentiating nursing diagnosis from medical diagnosis promote improved health care services and outcomes?
>
> Is confidence in APN diagnosing related to confidence in decision-making and critical thinking expertise?
>
> What kind of diagnostic capability should be emphasised in advanced nursing practice?
>
> Will extending the authority for nurses to order and interpret diagnostic testing enhance health care services?

The discussion of the use of nursing diagnosis versus medical diagnosis in advanced nursing practice can be controversial, and some practice acts reserve diagnosis to physicians. One view of diagnosis is that it is basically informed decision-making provided by a health care professional with and on behalf of a patient or family. In the drive toward seamless or comprehensive health care services for the world's populations, it would seem beneficial that the skill of appropriate diagnosis and related patient management be considered as universal aspects of practice, rather than belonging to a single body of professionals.

The debate can be related to the desire by nursing educators and leaders, as well as medicine, to clearly define or place limitations on scope for advanced nursing practice. Advanced nursing practice may be unduly restricted where the right to make a 'medical diagnosis' falls completely in the domain of medicine.

Reaction to nurse diagnosing in the United States has changed since the beginnings of advanced practice. The extension of nursing skills within hospital settings was in keeping with what other professionals had associated with nursing, even though nurses were practising at a more advanced level. For instance, in response to rapidly increasing technological advances, nurses in coronary care units (CCU) developed diagnostic and other technical skills alongside physician colleagues. This simultaneous skill enrichment contributed to collegial relationships and collaboration. The CCU nurses 'blurred the invisible boundary separating the disciplines of nursing and medicine. They were diagnosing and treating.' (Keeling & Bigbee, 2005, p. 22)

In the United States, as the NP role and related nursing education developed and adopted a medical model for diagnosing, the view emerged that NPs were 'essentially stepping over the invisible medical boundary' into the sphere of influence associated with 'curing', a domain claimed by physicians (Keeling & Bigbee, 2005, p. 23). This use of medical terminology by NPs for diagnosing caused medical practitioners to see this as intrusion into medical practice, while at the same time nursing leaders and educators viewed this as a move away from the nursing model.

In the United Kingdom, although Walsh (2001) points out that diagnosis 'is working out what is wrong with the patient and giving it a label' (p. 8), nurses tended to oppose inclusion of this concept in nursing functions as the use of the word diagnosis was associated only with physicians. McGee (2003) favours an emphasis on nursing diagnosis and intervention in order to enhance the scope of nursing practice rather than encouraging nurses to take on medical roles.

Just as nurse prescribing provokes a controversy, the issue of diagnosing also points to the need for considerable deliberation. It is the view of the authors that if consistency of care is a goal for health services, using a common diagnostic language is one way to attain this goal.

Approaching APN diagnosing

Questions to consider and discuss when deciding on the diagnostic role of the APN include:

(1) Is the topic of APN diagnosis controversial?
(2) If it is controversial, what are the reasons given for not permitting, or restricting the diagnostic role of the APN?
(3) What are the advantages of including diagnosis in APN responsibilities?

(4) Is there language in any of the existing professional practice acts or regulations that defines differences in medical diagnosis and nursing diagnosis?
(5) Will restrictive definitions of diagnosing impact or limit the kind and quality of services provided by the APN?

Hospital privileges

> Why should APNs have the authority to admit and discharge from health facilities?
>
> How will having this privilege influence delivery of care?
>
> What factors will influence granting this authority to nurses?

Hospital privileges, or the ability to admit and discharge from a health facility, have traditionally been associated with physicians in most areas of the world. This is being challenged as recognition grows that these policies have the potential to compromise the efficient and effective delivery of care. The term 'hospital privileges' originated from the process of awarding a status to physicians who had successfully completed a hospital's screening process. With the increasing tendency to adopt a business perspective to health care, and a growing desire of hospitals to maximise occupancy rates, there is now an opportunity for APNs to consider acquiring privileges for admitting and discharging patients from health facilities (Buppert, 2004).

APNs can provide services in primary heath care (PHC) without hospital privileges as long as arrangements are made for hospitalisation to be taken care of by an appropriate provider. Advanced practice nurses employed within hospital settings and who work on hospital wards in specialty roles are unlikely to see this as a relevant practice issue. However, while the urgency of this matter is not high in the present international health agenda, the dynamic nature of health care could make the provision of hospital privileges an issue for APNs. Health authorities may find it advantageous to accord this privilege to certain nurses.

Approaching APN hospital privileges

Questions to consider and discuss with respect to hospital privileges for the APN include:

(1) Does the APN require hospital privileges to provide continuity of care?
(2) If the advanced nursing practice role does not include admission and discharge from the hospital, is there a method to facilitate this in a way that best serves patient needs?
(3) Are there practices and regulations in place that prohibit APN hospital privileges?

Domains of practice

Read & Roberts-Davis (2000) from their study of CNS and NP models present in the United Kingdom between 1996 and 1998 provide examples of domains of clinical practice (Table 2.2). Conclusions from the study indicate that the main difference between these roles is that the NP is a generalist who conducts assessments in undifferentiated conditions, while the CNS practices within a specialist area where an initial diagnosis has already been made. This explanation provides a way to begin to discuss the various dimensions of NP versus CNS practice, or the alternatives of hospital-based versus PHC-based advanced nursing practice roles.

The Canadian Nurses Association (2002) framework for advanced nursing practice states that the nature of practice is based on characteristics and competencies rather than domain or practice setting. In addition, the complexity of these nursing roles is related to not only clinical practice but also to the education,

Table 2.2 Domains of practice. (Source: Adapted from Read and Roberts-Davis, 2000, with permission.)

CNS Domains of Clinical Activity	
Condition Specific Domain (differentiated)	Examples of specialty care: Breast, Stoma, Diabetes, Cardiac, Haematology, Gynaecology, Urology, Oncology, Drug Dependency, etc.
Area Specific Domain (differentiated)	Examples: Intensive Care Unit, Coronary Care Unit, Orthopaedic Unit, Nurse Managed Community Hospitals and related services
Client Group Specific Domain (differentiated)	Examples: Elderly Mentally Ill. Adolescent Mental Health, Children or Gerontological Specialist
NP Domains of Clinical Activity	
Client Group Specific Domain (undifferentiated)	Examples: Homeless, Travellers, Children or Gerontological Specialist (generic)
Area Specific Domain (undifferentiated)	Examples: Accident & Emergency, Minor Injuries Clinic
Community Clinical Nursing Domain (undifferentiated)	Examples: Family or General Practice/Primary Care Nursing, Occupational Health
Public Health Nursing Domain	Examples: School Health, Public Health Visiting

research or administration aspects of the role. Even though New Zealand has chosen the NP title, the Nursing Council of New Zealand (2002) and the New Zealand Ministry of Health (MOHNZ, 2002) documents refer to a CNS as an expert nurse specialising in a field of practice. Roodbol (2005) when promoting professional collaboration between physicians and APNs in the Netherlands writes that there is only 'one domain: that is the domain of the patient' (p. 4).

In comparing the CNS to the NP roles, the specialised nature of the CNS is set against the more comprehensive practice usually associated with the NP. Read & Roberts-Davis (2000) noted that difficulty arises when CNS and NP operate under different titles. It seems that it is not possible to assume from title that reference is being made to the same type of APN, as currently there appears to be a trend for the CNS to take on NP-type roles, and for NP to incorporate more specialisation into their practice.

In describing CNS practice in the United States, the National Association of Clinical Nurse Specialists (NACNS, 2005) agree with Read & Roberts-Davis (2000) in describing the CNS as an expert clinician in a specialised area of practice identified in terms of population, setting, disease or medical subspecialty, type of care or type of problem. Heitkemper and Bond (2004) when reviewing CNS history in the United States note that intensive care units have been a traditional site for this role. These authors also comment that even when the CNS role includes health promotion and disease prevention activities, they are specialty-based e.g. diabetes care, pain management, heart failure, wound healing and stress management.

Although NP practice in the United States tends to be associated with primary health care there are practice areas and sites considered to be NP specialties that are hospital-based such as the acute care nurse practitioner (Hravnak *et al.*, 2005) or blended CNS and NP roles that include settings ranging from primary health to tertiary care (Skalla *et al.*, 2005). A lengthy experience with advanced nursing practice in the United States has not appeared to increase clarity as to specificity regarding domains of advanced nursing practice.

To meet societal demands and developing health care needs requiring specialised nursing care with a higher level of knowledge, the concept of the APN was introduced as a nursing specialisation in Bahrain, Hong Kong, Switzerland, Thailand and Taiwan. However, there is no common distinguishable definition of these roles, title use remains unclear, and the scope of practice has yet to be distinctly defined. In countries such as Australia, Canada and the United States differences in terminology use among states and provinces adds to the confusion. Thus it is difficult to assess if progress toward advanced practice is being made or if what is occurring is simply a change in titling with no or little alteration in scope of practice. In the hope of avoiding this confusion the Philippines has developed a national model based from the beginning on progressive and specific criteria defining the specialist role. The criteria specify the increasing depth of knowledge and clinical experience required to move from Certified Nurse Clinician I and II to the CNS role (Professional Regulation Commission, Board of Nursing, Manila, 2002; key informant, personal communication).

Table 2.3 Practice domains connected to clinical settings. (Source: Key Informants, personal communication.)

Country	Setting	Domain of Practice
Australia	PHC	Comprehensive Services, Community, Rural and Remote
Bahrain	Hospitals PHC	Specialty: Cardiac, Mental Health, Emergency, Maternity Community Health Home Care
Botswana	PHC	Comprehensive Services
Canada	Hospitals	Specialty: Specific Age-based Patient Populations, Specific Clinical Areas, Specific disease Processes, Specific Communities
	PHC	Comprehensive Services in Rural and Remote areas
Hong Kong	Hospital	Specialty: Diabetes, Wound/Ostomy, Cardiac, HIV/AIDS, Urology
Iceland	Hospital	Specialty: Paediatrics, Adult, Obstetric, Critical Care, Pain Management
Ireland	PHC	Comprehensive Services
Japan	Hospital	Specialty: PHC, Paediatrics, Adult Care, Mental Health, Elder Care
Macau	Hospital	Specialty: Critical Care Hospice/Palliative Care, Hemodialysis, Cardiovascular, Gynaecology/Obstetrics
Netherlands	Hospital	Specialty: Thoracic, Critical Care, Oncology, Paediatrics, Immunology
New Zealand	Hospital PHC General Practitioner Offices	Specialty: School, Home, Occupational, Neonatal, Maori Health, Ambulatory Care Comprehensive Services
Philippines	Hospital PHC	Specialty: Medical-Surgical, Mother/Child, Mental Health Community Services
Republic of South Africa	Hospital PHC	Specialty: Intensive Care, Operating Room, Occupational Health, Community Services Home Care
Singapore	Hospital	Specialty
Switzerland	Hospital	Specialty HIV/AIDS Services, Renal Transplant, Oncology, Pain Management, Families of Children with Cleft Lip/Palate
Taiwan	Hospital	Specialty: Adult Care, Elderly Care
United Kingdom	Hospital PHC General Practitioner Offices	Specialised across all Specialties Comprehensive Services
United States	Hospitals PHC	Specialised across all specialties Comprehensive Services
Western Pacific: Vanuatu, Kiribati, Samoa, Fiji, Cook	PHC	Comprehensive Services

Practice settings

Advanced practice nurses and NPs are establishing a presence as an integral part of the workforce in the United States, United Kingdom, Canada, New Zealand, Australia, Western Pacific and Botswana. In addition, countries in Africa, Southeast Asia, the Middle East and Europe are reporting initiatives, assessing pilot studies and implementing the basic concepts of advanced practice nursing in a variety of settings. Schober (2004b) emphasises that '. . . integrating advanced practice nursing into hospitals and primary health care settings has the potential for improving accessibility and advancing quality of care for patients and their families' (p. 2). Using practice settings that identify service provision by an APN is one way to dissociate the reliance on title or domain in classifying the role.

At a glance, whether by setting or practice domain, it is apparent that the global presence of APNs is extensive. As noted by other authors and researchers, titles, scope of practice and areas of practice are described in inconsistent ways throughout the world. One way to look at possibilities for advanced nursing practice is to connect the domains of practice to the physical facility, institution or site where practice takes place. An analysis done in this way has the potential for connecting provision of services to the needs of the setting. Table 2.3 provides some examples of the connection of settings to practice domains in various countries.

Conclusion

This chapter explored various facets of advanced nursing practice. The authors have highlighted important issues needing debate and discussion when considering the nature of the role. No single method or approach can be said to be sufficient to embrace all aspects of role development.

The information obtained from key informants, published and unpublished sources demonstrated how extraordinarily sensitive the characteristics of the APN role are to the context. As a result, the nature of advanced nursing practice in international settings is diverse, complex and dynamic. An international consensus on the nature of advanced nursing practice would assist countries by providing direction while allowing the role to be tailored to country needs and resource capabilities.

References

American Academy of Nurse Practitioners. (2002a). *Nurse practitioners as an advanced practice nurse.* Role position statement. Washington, D.C.: Author. Retrieved June 28, 2005 from http://www.aanp.org

American Academy of Nurse Practitioners. (2002b). *Scope of Practice for Nurse Practitioners.* Position paper. Washington, D.C.: Author. Retrieved June 28, 2005 from http://www.aanp.org

American Academy of Nurse Practitioners. (2002c). *Nurse practitioner prescriptive privilege*. Position paper. Washington, D.C.: Author. Retrieved June 28, 2005 from http://www.aanp.org

American Nurses Association. (1996). *Scope of practice and standards of advanced nursing practice*. Washington D.C.: Author.

Anthony, C.E., del Bueno, D. (1993). A performance-based development system. *Nurse Management*, **24**(6), 32–34.

Ballantyne, A., Cheek, J., O'Brien, B., Pincombe, J. (1998). Nursing competencies: Ground work in aged and extended care. *International Journal of Nursing Practice*, **4**(3), 156–165.

Bloom, B. (1956). *The taxonomy of educational objectives: Handbook 1*. London: Longman.

Bloom, B., Krathwohl, D.R., Masia, B.B. (1965). *The taxonomy of educational objectives: Handbook 2*. London: Longman.

Bowling, A., Stilwell, B. (1988). (Eds) *The nurse in family practice: Practice nurses and nurse practitioners in primary health care*. London: Scutari Press.

Brown, S.J. (1998). A framework for advanced practice nursing. *Journal of Professional Nursing*, **14**, 157–164.

Buchan, J., Calman, L. (2004a). *Implementing nurse prescribing: An updated review of current practice internationally*. Monograph 16, Geneva: ICN.

Buchan, J., Calman, L. (2004b). *Skill-mix and policy change in the health workforce: Nurses in advanced roles*, OECD Health Working Papers No. 17, DELSA/ELSA/WD/HEA, 8.

Buppert, C. (2004). *Nurse practitioner's business practice and legal guide*. Sudbury, MA: Jones and Bartlett Publishers.

Canadian Medical Association, Canadian Nurses Association, Canadian Pharmacists Association. (2003). *Scopes of practice: Joint position statement*. Retrieved 5 October, 2005 from http://www.cna-aiic.ca/CNA/issues/position/practice/default_e.aspx

Canadian Nurses Association. (2002). *Advanced nursing practice: A national framework*. Ottawa: Author.

Carryer, J. (2002). Nurse practitioners: an evolutionary role. *Kai Taiki Nursing New Zealand*, **8**(10), 23.

Castledine, G. (1996). The role and criteria of an advanced practice nurse practitioner. *British Journal of Nursing*, **5**(5): 288–289.

Castledine, G. (2002). The important aspects of nurse specialist roles, Castledine Column, *British Journal of Nursing*, **11**(5).

Castledine, G. (2003). The development of advanced nursing practice in the UK. In P. McGee, G. Castledine (Eds). *Advanced nursing practice*, 2nd Edition, pp. 8–16, Oxford: Blackwell Publishing.

Cattini, P., Knowles, V. (1999). Core competencies for clinical nurse specialists: a usable framework. *Journal of Clinical Nursing*, **8**(5), 505–511.

Chan, U.W. (2001). *Professional nursing and nurse specialists in Hong Kong and Macau*. Revista de Ciencias da Sude de Macau, Macao: Servicos de Saude de Macau. September 2001.

Coleman, S., Fox, J. (2003). Clinical practice benchmarking and advanced practice. In P. McGee & G. Castledine (Eds), *Advanced Nursing Practice*, 2nd Edition, pp. 47–58. Oxford: Blackwell Publishing.

Daly, W., Carnwell, R. (2003). Nursing roles and levels of practice: a framework for differentiating between elementary, specialist and advanced nursing practice. *Journal of Clinical Nursing*, **12**(2), 158–167.

del Bueno, D.J. (1995a). Spotlight on . . . Ready, willing, able? Staff competence in the workplace. *Journal of Nursing Administration*, **25**(9), 14–16.

del Bueno, D.J. (1995b). Why can't new grads think like nurses? *Nurse Educator*, **19**(4), 9–11.

Dunning, T. (2002). *Comments re: A draft for the nurse practitioner/advanced practice nurse scope of advanced practice for ICN*. Unpublished.

Gardner, G., Carryer, J., Dunn, S., Gardner, A. (2004). *Nurse Practitioner Standards Project: Report to Australian Nursing Council.* Australian Nursing Council: Author.

Girot, E. (2000). Assessment of graduates and diplomats in practice in the UK – are we measuring the same level of competence? *Journal of Clinical Nursing,* **9**: 330–337.

Goolsby, M.J., Towers, J., Dempster, J.S. (2005). *Trends in U.S. nurse practitioner practice: A 15-year comparison of a vital health care discipline.* Presentation at the ICN 23rd Quadrennial Congress, Taipei, Taiwan.

Guilbert, J. (1987). *Educational handbook for health personnel.* Geneva: World Health Organization.

Hamric, A.B. (1996). A definition of advanced practice nursing. In A.B. Hamric, J.A. Spross, C.M. Hanson (Eds), *Advanced nursing practice: An integrative approach,* pp. 25–41. Philadelphia: W.B. Saunders.

Hamric, A.B. (2005). A definition of advanced practice nursing. In A.B. Hamric, J.A. Spross, C.M. Hanson (Eds) *Advanced nursing practice: An integrative approach,* pp. 85–108. St. Louis: Elsevier Saunders.

Hanson, C.M. (2005). Understanding regulatory, legal and credentialing requirements. In A.B. Hamric, J.A. Spross, C.M. Hanson (Eds) *Advanced practice nursing: An integrative approach,* pp. 781–808. St. Louis: Elsevier Saunders.

Hravnak, M., Kleinpell, R.M., Magdic, K.M., Guttendorf, J. (2005). The acute care nurse practitioner. In A.B. Hamric, J.A. Spross, C.M. Hanson (Eds) *Advanced practice nursing: An integrative approach,* pp. 475–514. St. Louis: Elsevier Saunders.

Heitkemper, M.M., Bond, E.F. (2004). Clinical nurse specialists: state of the profession and challenges ahead. *Clinical Nurse Specialist,* **18**(3): 135–140.

International Council of Nurses. (1997). *An approval system for schools of nursing. Guidelines.* Geneva, Author.

International Council of Nurses. (2002). *Definition and characteristics of the role.* Retrieved June 21, 2005 from http://www.icn-apnetwork.org

International Council of Nurses. (2003a). *ICN framework of competencies for the generalist nurse.* Geneva: Author.

International Council of Nurses. (2003b). *ICN framework and core competencies for the family nurse.* Geneva: Author.

International Council of Nurses. (2005). *Scope, standards and competencies for advanced practice nursing.* Final working draft. Retrieved October 25, 2005 from http://www.icn-apnetwork.org

Jamieson, J.R. (1993). Competency-based professional standards: A fundamental consideration. *Journal of Manipulative and Physiologica; Therapeutics,* **16**(7): 498–504.

Keeling, A.W., Bigbee, J.L. (2005). The history of advanced practice in the United States, in A.B. Hamric, J.A. Spross, C.M. Hanson (Eds) *Advanced practice nursing: an integrative approach,* pp. 3–45. St. Louis: Elsevier Saunders.

Klein, T.A. (2005). Scope of practice and the nurse practitioner: regulation, competency, expansion, and evolution. *Topics in Advanced Practice Nursing eJournal,* **5**(2): 2005. Retrieved June 28, 2005 from www.medscape.com/viewpublication/527_index

Krathwohl, D.R., Bloom, B.S., Masia, B.B. (1956). *Taxonomy of educational objectives: The classification of educational goals.* Handbook II: Affective Domain. New York: Longman.

Lenburg, C.B. (1999a). Redesigning expectations for initial and continuing competence for contemporary nursing practice. *Online Journal of Issues in Nursing.* Retrieved October 25, 2005 from http://www.nursingworld.org/ojin/topic10/tpc10_1

Lenburg, C.B. (1999b). The framework, concepts and methods of the competency, outcomes and performance assessment (COPA) model. *Online Journal of Issues in Nursing.* Retrieved October 25, 2005 from http://www.nursingworld.org/ojin/topic10/tpc10_2.htm

Maclaine, K., Walsh, M., Harston, B. (2004). *Embracing nurse practitioners within the post-registration regulatory framework.* Submission for Post-Registration Review Conference.

McAllister, M. (1998). Competency standards clarifying the issues. *Contemporary Nurse,* 7(3): 131–137.

McGee, P. (2003). Advanced health assessment. In P. McGee, G. Castledine (Eds) *Advanced Nursing Practice,* 2nd Edition, pp. 85–97. Oxford: Blackwell Publishing.

Ministry of Health, New Zealand. (2002). *Nurse practitioners in New Zealand.* Wellington: MOHNZ.

National Association of Clinical Nurse Specialists. (2005). *Scope of practice for the CNS,* Organizational web site, Retrieved June 30, 2005 from www.nacns.org

National Council for the Professional Development of Nursing and Midwifery. (2001; 2004 2nd Edition) *Framework for the advanced nurse practitioner and advanced midwife practitioner posts.* Dublin: Author.

National Organization of Nurse Practitioner Faculties [NONPF]. (2000). *Domains and competencies of nurse practitioner practice.* Washington, D.C.: Author.

National Organization of Nurse Practitioner Faculties [NONPF]. (2002). *Nurse practitioner primary competencies in specialty areas: Adult, family, gerontological, pediatric, and women's health.* Washington, D.C.: Author.

New Zealand Gazette. (2004). *Scope of practice – nurse practitioner.* No. 120, p. 2959. Wellington: NCNZ.

Nursing Council of New Zealand. (2002). *The nurse practitioner: Responding to health needs in New Zealand,* 3rd Edition. Wellington: Author.

Perry, L. (1997). Critical incidents, crucial issues: insights into the working lives of registered nurses. *Journal of Clinical Nursing,* **6**, 131–137.

Professional Regulation Commission, Board of Nursing, Manila. (2002). *Nursing Speciality Certification Program. BON Res. No.14S. 1999 and Guidelines for Implementation,* BON Res. No. 118 – S2002. Manila: Author.

Read, S., Roberts-Davis, M. (2000). *Preparing nurse practitioners for the 21st century.* Executive summary from the report of the project Realizing specialist and advanced nursing practice: establishing the parameters of and identifying the competencies for 'nurse practitioner' roles and evaluating programmes of preparation (RSANP). University of Sheffield: Author. Full report available at http://www.shef.ac.uk/snm/research/prepnp/index.html

Roberts-Davis, M., Read, S. (2001). Clinical role clarification: using the Delphi method to establish similarities and differences between nurse practitioners and clinical nurse specialists. *Journal of Clinical Nursing,* **10**(1), 33–43.

Roodbol, P. (2005). *Willing o'-the-wisps, stumbling runs, toll roads and song lines: study into the structural rearrangement of tasks between nurses and physicians.* Summary of doctoral dissertation. Unpublished.

Royal College of Nursing. (July 2002, revised March 2005). *Nurse practitioners – an RCN guide to the nurse practitioner role, competencies and programme approval.* London: Author.

Schober, M. (2004a). Advanced practice nursing: perspectives and challenges. *Nursing Excellence in Transactions* [NET], 8th Issue. Hong Kong: Queen Elizabeth Hospital, Central Nursing Division.

Schober, M. (2004b). Global perspective on advanced practice. In L. Joel (Ed.) *Advanced practice nursing: Essentials for role development.* Philadelphia: F.A. Davis.

Seitio, O.S. (2000). *The family nurse practitioner in Botswana: issues and challenges.* Presented at the 8th International NP Conference, San Diego, Ca. Retrieval option www.icn-apnetwork.org

Skalla, K., Hamric, A., Caron, A. (2005). The blended role of the clinical nurse specialist and nurse practitioner. In A.B. Hamric, J.A. Spross, C.M. Hanson (Eds) *Advanced practice nursing: an integrative approach,* pp. 515–550. St. Louis: Elsevier Saunders.

Spross, J.A., Lawson, M.T. (2005). Conceptualization of advanced practice nursing. In A.B. Hamric, J.A. Spross, C.M. Hanson (Eds) *Advanced practice nursing: an integrative approach.* pp. 47–84. St. Louis: Elsevier Saunders.

Towers, J. (January 2005). After forty years. *Journal of the American Academy of Nurse Practitioners,* **17**(1), 9–13.

Turris, S.A., Smith, S., Gillrie, C. (2005). *Nurse practitioners in the ED: a rebuttal.* CJEM/JCMU **7**(3), 147–148, Letters.

Uys, L.R. (2004). *Competency in nursing.* Geneva: World Health Organization. Retrieved October 25 2005 from http://rsdesigns.com/extranet/IMG/pdf/Competency_in_Nursing.pdf#search='Competency%20in%20Nursing%20uys'

Walsh, M. (2001). The nurse practitioner role in hospital: professional and organisational issues. In M. Walsh, A. Crumbie, S. Revely (Eds) *Nurse practitioners clinical skills and professional issues.* Oxford: Butterworth-Heinemann.

Watson, R., Stimpson, A., Topping, A., Porock, D. (2002). Clinical competence assessment in nursing: a systematic review of the literature. *Journal of Advanced Nursing*, **39**(5): 421–431.

World Health Organization. (2001a). *Department of Essential Drugs and Medicines Policy: Essential drugs in brief.* No. 5. Geneva: Author.

World Health Organization. (2001b). *National drug policies.* http://www.who.int/m/topics/national_drug_policies/en/index.html

World Health Organization-Eastern Mediterranean Region [WHO-EMRO]. (2001). *Report on the fifth meeting of the regional advisory panel on nursing and consultation on advanced practice nursing and nurse prescribing: implications for regulation, nursing education and practice in the Eastern Mediterranean.* Cairo: Author.

World Health Organization-Western Pacific Region [WHO-WPRO]. (2001). *Mid-level and nurse practitioners in the Pacific: Models and issues.* Manila: Author.

Chapter 3
Role and practice development

Introduction

In the process of defining the potential for the advancement of nursing, key stakeholders may have the authority to promote, block or ignore developments in advances in nursing. Depending on country or locale this could be the ministries and departments of health, national health agencies, hospital authorities, health administrators, educational institutions, regulators or professional associations, and an increasingly informed public. Pivotal decisions may be in the hands of authorities with limited understanding of health care, nursing or advanced practice issues. Thus it is important that knowledgeable policy makers and nursing leaders have the opportunity to facilitate informed decision-making and promote effective strategies.

This chapter aims to provide information, examples, and models to consider during the process of assessing the environment when introducing and implementing advanced nursing practice roles.

Striving for the ideal: transitional processes

Initiatives associated with launching advanced nursing practice roles arise from varied factors and are often unpredictable in the manner in which they evolve. The introduction of advanced nursing practice involves a process which includes careful consideration of what models and frameworks may be suitably adapted, as well as a careful analysis of the interest and motives for implementing these new roles. Confident, motivated and committed advocates for nursing advancement may be as important as pursuing a sequential path through a predetermined process. Concepts, suggestions and strategies described in this section are intended to explain some of the factors that influence the process of change, and provide a basis for successful planning when introducing advanced nursing practice into a health system or facility.

Some critical questions that need to be debated in the early stages include:

> What is it that has to be changed to introduce advanced nursing practice?
>
> How do you go about making the change?
>
> Why is the change needed or beneficial?
>
> Who will benefit by the change?
>
> Who should participate in the transitional and implementation process?

Buchan and Calman (2004) in a report examining the evidence on role change and delegation from physicians to advanced practice nurses (APN), nurse practitioners (NP) and nurses in hospital settings and primary health care (PHC), indicate that evidence supports the view that nurses can provide care at least equivalent to doctors in defined situations. This report also points to the emergence of the visible and complex contributions made by advanced nursing in improving the quality of health care. Reports from key informants (personal communication), international experience and observations during site visits made by the authors along with unpublished narratives and reports support this contention.

Despite extensive literature available to support these nursing roles, it is unclear what kind of process is needed to shape new role development, and how possible it is to adapt models in current use in countries with established APN roles to new situations. Scrutiny of research on APN roles indicates that a substantial number of the published studies are descriptive commentary, while others have procedural weaknesses. Most published analytical studies have been undertaken in the United States, with notable contributions from Canada and the United Kingdom and more recently Australia and New Zealand. Their relevance to other countries and health care systems is unclear (Buchan and Dal Poz, 2002; Gardner *et al.*, 2004).

Whatever approach is taken, no matter which model or framework is considered for adaptation and regardless of the strengths or challenges accompanying consideration of advanced nursing roles, change is unavoidable if they are to be introduced. Change initiatives often start with great enthusiasm and visible support, which then can deteriorate before the goal is reached. Sometimes this is due to delays in implementation; sometimes attention or commitment of professionals and stakeholders wavers; or possibly day-to-day issues and priorities interfere. The initiative may lack the necessary level of agreement or a clear articulation of the benefits to support the need for change (Heifitz, 1993). In striving for the ideal model, framework or strategies, stakeholders enter a process of progressive development. While striving to adapt the APN role to a new context, pioneers may face multiple challenges, continually having to debate the issues, justify the changes and refine conclusions and proposals for action.

Assessing the opportunities and need for advanced nursing practice

> What factors need to be considered in assessing the value of having advanced practice nurses as part of the healthcare workforce?
>
> Will introduction of new initiatives be associated with workforce and service needs or advancement of the nursing profession?
>
> Who will organise, support and evaluate development?

There may be no identifiable common starting point when it comes to deciding whether to introduce APN roles. Multiple considerations may come together to raise awareness and interest in concepts and principles associated with advanced nursing practice. Factors such as availability of human and financial resources, the regulatory context, culture, language, customs and traditions are likely to influence interest and success in implementing new nursing roles. From the perspective of policy, organisational structure and countrywide systems, advanced nursing practice may be one of several options being considered by decision-makers seeking solutions for populations needing or requesting services (Buchan & Calman, 2004). This section will suggest some ways for exploring the context and developing appropriate strategies for role implementation. Illustrations describing how various countries have approached this task are also given.

Scanning the environment

If you are planning to introduce the APN role into your organisation or health system, change or strengthen existing roles (e.g. change in scope of practice, obtain title protection, or introduce credentialing) you may find that scanning your environment will assist you to think strategically as well as be more purposeful and realistic in planning your actions to reach intended goals.

Environmental scanning is the acquisition and use of information about events, trends and relationships in the environment, the knowledge of which would assist you to plan a course of action. The results help to provide the context for your action.

There are many ways to carry out an environmental scan. The authors propose two simple techniques that ICN (2005) has found useful when working with nurse leaders.

Stakeholder analysis

Stakeholders are individuals, groups or organisations who have an impact on, or are affected by, what you are proposing to do. It will help you to make your planning decisions if you can find out (a) who they are, (b) what their interest (or stake) is, and (c) what assumptions you hold about them. Remember that you will want to scan those who oppose or are undecided, as well as supporters. A stakeholder analysis should always be done at the beginning of a project.

Primary stakeholders are those who are ultimately affected, that is those who expect to benefit from or be adversely affected by the intervention. For example, health service users, especially those who will be accessing APN services, policy and decision-makers at the Ministry of Health, other health professionals, the professional associations, regulators, health professions and educators, the institutions preparing health care providers, and institutions or other clinical settings where they will be practising. Secondary stakeholders are groups with some intermediary role such as the departments of finance at the ministries of health and education, potential funders for developing APN roles, and health service planners.

Stakeholder analysis aims to:

- Identify and define the characteristics of potential key stakeholders
- Assess the manner in which they might affect, or be affected by, the proposal related to advanced practice development
- Understand the relations between stakeholders (i.e. how does the stakeholder regard the others you have on your list?), including an assessment of the real or potential conflicts of interest and expectation of stakeholders
- Assess the capacity of different stakeholders to participate in or obstruct the goals of the proposal
- Establish what resources the stakeholder will wish to commit (or avoid committing) to the project (Overseas Development Administration, 1995).

One of the important areas to evaluate is the degree of influence or power which stakeholders may have to control or persuade others into making decisions, taking certain actions, facilitating implementation, or exerting influence which affects the evolution of the advanced nursing negatively. This power may lie in the ability to command and control decision-making, the budget or access to strategic resources; and authority derived from leadership (formal and informal, charisma, political, familial or through connections to influential persons).

Other stakeholders may be those who may have few powers of influence, but to whom developing advanced nursing practice is important. For example it may be the groups whom the APN will serve, or members of the profession who regard development of advanced nursing practice as being important to the future of the profession, and its ability to meet growing health care needs.

As a minimum the stakeholder analysis should enable you to do the following:

- Identify (a) whom you want to enlist to help and work with as an ally; (b) who may block or hinder you reaching your goals, and why. Knowing your opponents as well as your allies helps you to prepare to respond to their concerns.
- Think about whether strategic alliances need to be developed, or if specific people need to be appointed to manage some relationships. You may find allies in a poorly served group who will benefit from the services of APNs; or researchers with data to support your case; or a government seeking to reform health services and which is ready to challenge traditional roles of health care providers. Opponents may be other nursing groups; other health professionals; a ministry of health reluctant to re-negotiate roles; budget holders (from the health or educational sectors) unwilling to commit the necessary resources.

For more detailed guidance on carrying out a stakeholder analysis the reader is recommended to consult *Guidance note on how to do stakeholder analysis of aid projects and programmes*, available at http://www.euforic.org/gb/stake1.htm.

SWOT analysis

A SWOT analysis is an effective way of identifying **S**trengths and **W**eaknesses (internal resources and capabilities), and for examining the **O**pportunities and **T**hreats factors (external to the organisation or situation). Strategies in an action plan are often better conceived when a well-done SWOT analysis has been carried out, and the results are used to build on strengths, eliminate or reduce weaknesses, and identify actions that can be done to minimise threats and create more opportunities.

A number of actions can be taken to improve the results of a SWOT analysis:

- The first key step is to be clear on what you are doing and why. The purpose of conducting a SWOT may be wide or narrow, general or specific. For example, you may be carrying out the SWOT prior to defining a national scope of practice for advanced nursing practice.
- Select appropriate contributors who will be knowledgeable about the issues that relate to the SWOT topic.
- Information on strengths and weaknesses should focus on the internal factors of skills, resources and assets, or lack of them. Opportunities and threats should focus on the external factors over which you have little or no control, such as social or economic factors. Weaknesses and threats can

constrain your actions, and must be made explicit and dealt with to facilitate action.

- There may be an exploratory stage when those you have asked to assist with the SWOT are asked to gather data in specific areas. This is followed by bringing all the participants together and collecting data on the four areas. The final step should be to ask each participant to select the five most important factors in each of the areas from those listed during the group process (See Figure 3.1 for helpful tips when undertaking a SWOT analysis).

Figure 3.2 indicates the type of strategies that you may consider based on the SWOT analysis (The Community Tool Box, undated). They can be summarised as:

Strength–Opportunity strategies pursue opportunities that are a good fit with the strengths you have identified. For example:

Strength: faculty capable of teaching at the level required for APN education.
Opportunity: health system reform is occurring.

Weakness–Opportunity use strategies that overcome weaknesses by pursuing opportunities. For example:

Weakness: lack nurses to provide clinical precepting; strength practice models.
Opportunity: funds available to acquire external resources to provide quality preceptorship who participate in preparing national staff for the APN role.

- Carry out the SWOT as a group process bringing together those you think have good knowledge of the internal and external contexts. Select a good facilitator for the exercise.
- Create an atmosphere conductive to the free flow of information so that participants can say what they feel to be appropriate, free from blame. The facilitator has a key role and should allow time for free flow of thought, but not too much. Do not allow the SWOT to become a blame-laying exercise.
- Start with strengths. Make sure that all ideas are real strengths, and not opportunities. They may relate to the group under analysis (in this case APNs and their practice), to the environment, to perceptions, and to people (e.g. skills, capabilities and knowledge).
- When listing weaknesses avoid making this an opportunity to focus on the negative but encourage an honest appraisal of the way things are (e.g. what obstacles may impede progress, what may need strengthening, where are the weak links). You may arrive at weaknesses that contradict strengths already identified. If after discussion you are unable to solve the contradictions, you should leave the question open, and plan to return later for final resolution.
- Opportunities give you the possibility of assessing the socio-economic, environmental, health systems and demographic factors, among others, and to evaluate the benefits. Do not lose sight of external influences and trends. You may also identify opportunities by looking at your strengths and asking yourself whether these open up any new avenues for action.
- Record all thoughts and ideas in the early stages, and be more selective in the final evaluation.
- Do not ignore the SWOT outcomes during the planning process.

Figure 3.1 Tips for carrying out a SWOT.

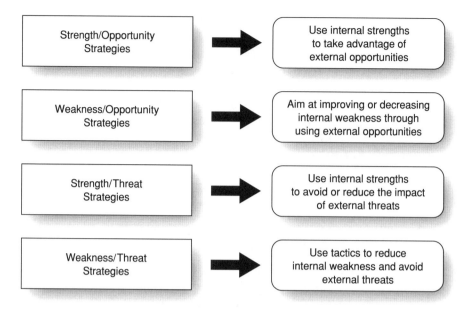

Figure 3.2 Strategies based on SWOT analysis. (Source: Community Tool Box. We encourage the reproduction of this material but ask that you credit the Community Tool Box: http//ctb.ku.edu/.)

Strength–Threat strategies identify the way strengths are used to overcome vulnerability to threats. For example:

Strengths: consumer groups are strong supporters of introducing advanced practice roles into the health system.
Weakness: decision–making is dominated by medicine.

Weakness–Threat strategies establish a defensive plan to prevent weaknesses increasing susceptibility to threats. For example:

Weakness: advanced practice nurses have not been integrated as part of the permanent government health human resources plan.
Threat: oversupply of physicians.
An example of a SWOT based on information from key informants (personal communication) is given in Appendix 3.

Introducing and supporting advanced nursing practice

In 1996, the Board of Nursing in the Philippines (BON) created a task force to facilitate the introduction of specialist nurses at the advanced level. Following two years of review of literature, internal and external expert consultation, dialogue, conferences and series of meetings, a position paper was submitted to the

BON recommending the creation of a Nursing Specialty Certification Council. The main task of the Council would be to accredit specialty organisations and certify nurses who meet the criteria for certification. At the time the proposal was submitted, no university-level clinical nurse specialist (CNS) programmes existed. Instrumental in constructively facing opposition from numerous sources was a nurse leader who demonstrated the need for a nurse specialist programme. This country initiative is in an early stage of development (Professional Regulation Commission, Board of Nursing, Manila, 2002; key informant, personal communication).

The Canadian Nurse Practitioner Initiative (CNPI, 2005) is funded through the Primary Health Care Transition Fund, and is therefore government supported. The purpose of this project is to develop the foundation for a shared national understanding of the role of NPs in PHC. Activities to achieve the initiative objectives include Canada-wide stakeholder consultations, literature reviews, focus groups and workshops. The national initiative running from 2004–2006 promoted collaboration amongst government staff, regulatory bodies, professional associations, NPs and educators. The CNPI aims to develop:

- A definition of the NP role
- Recommendations for collaborative practice models
- Recommendations for curriculum design
- Recruitment, retention and deployment strategies
- Recommendations for legislation and regulation
- A national licensure examination
- Processes to support professional mobility
- Strategies to reduce barriers to practice
- A communications and marketing plan to promote the NP role.

The Government of New Zealand, while recognising nurses were already providing some services at an advanced level, established a task-force in 1998 to identify 'the barriers that prevent nursing from improving the service to its patients' (p 5). The task-force examined strategies to remove those barriers and release the unused nursing potential. The Government adopted the recommendations of the task-force, amongst which was the need to regulate advanced nursing practice. In this example of a strategy for implementing the APN role, the presence of a supportive Chief Nursing Advisor at the Ministry of Health was critical to the success achieved in obtaining government recognition that regulation, formal recognition and employment of APNs would improve health outcomes of the population. The Nursing Council of New Zealand (NCNZ, 2002) working with the Ministry of Health defined two clear areas of work:

- Consultation and policy development around the title, education standards and competencies
- Policy development around prescribing, including mechanisms to regulate prescribing, establish education standards, curricula and competencies.

The Ministry also focused on enacting the necessary legislative changes to allow prescribing. Action was taken to remove other barriers to advanced practice by facilitating employment and finding funding for nurse practitioner positions. As of June 2005, New Zealand had registered 15 nurse practitioners in the fields of neonatal nursing, mental health, wound care, primary health, diabetes and related conditions, child health and aged care (Ministry of Health New Zealand, 2002; NCNZ, 2002; key informants, personal communication).

Singapore, in order to develop advanced nursing roles, looked at practice in the United States, United Kingdom, Australia and New Zealand and decided that its preference was an approach complementary to physician practice. In 2001, a committee comprising nurse leaders and physicians began to examine how to implement advanced nursing practice. The Nursing Branch of the Ministry of Health worked with the Division of Graduate Medical Studies and the National University of Singapore to develop advanced nursing practice programmes with a clinical focus. In July 2004, two APN interns began to practise in the emergency medicine and breast cancer areas (Ang, 2002; key informant, personal communication).

Adopting a national strategy from the beginning seems to promote cohesiveness and consistency contributing to smoother implementation of advanced nursing practice services. National efforts may begin when APN interest first arises, or may be a result of trying to consolidate a number of unrelated developments already in place. Some of the initiatives described are too new, and the numbers of APNs produced are too small in number, to allow definitive analysis of the outcomes of these strategies. However, the fact that they have survived and reached some definitive goals makes them useful approaches to consider in strategy development.

Innovative and new health care services provided by non-physician health workers are commonly introduced where there is a physician shortage, when doctors have a busy practice and are unable to keep up with the workload, or to staff services where it has proved difficult to recruit physicians. Health care reform that focuses on transfer of public hospital patients to the private sector, or the shift of health care from hospitals to community settings presents further possibilities for advanced nursing practice. An urgent need to improve coverage and access to health care services can substantiate the case for introducing new or changed health provider roles. Offering the advanced nursing practice option when key stakeholders are exploring alternatives to fill gaps in service delivery carries a greater likelihood of success.

Some of the reasons given by key informants (personal communication) for introducing advanced nursing practice roles in various countries are shown in Table 3.1. They are various, but the growth of advanced nursing practice in several of the reporting countries relate to the need to improve access to PHC, to solve a physician shortage, and to respond to an increased demand for nurse specialists. What emerges is that solving how to meet urgent health care needs in the presence of a physician shortage usually requires an immediate strategy as was adopted in Timor-Leste where a six-month Advanced Practice

Table 3.1 Identified reasons by country for introducing APN roles. (Source: Key Informants, personal communication.)

Country	Reason(s) given for introducing APNs
Australia	Shortage of doctors, especially in rural and remote areas Nursing desire for a clinical ladder
Bahrain	Demand for specialised nursing care
Botswana	Urgent need for PHC services
Canada	Need for access to PHC services Increased emphasis on health promotion & disease prevention Emphasis on team care delivery Public demand
Hong Kong	Education programme development Change in nursing grade to improve clinical focus
Iceland	Exposure/education out of country Rising need for specialist nursing services
Ireland	Access to PHC services Career path tied to pay scale
Japan	Need for highly skilled specialty nurses
Macau	Consumer demand for quality services Inspiration of nursing professionals Privatisation of services
Netherlands	Shortage of doctors and nurses Hospital need for services Career advancement
New Zealand	Standardisation of current and new nursing roles
Pakistan	Education programme development
Philippines	Progression of specialisation in nursing
Singapore	Progression of specialty and subspecialty nursing
Sweden	Identified population with need: elderly Education programme development
Switzerland	Education programme development Knowledge advancement for nurses Anticipated physician shortage
Taiwan	Physician shortage Increasing inpatient acuity
Thailand	PHC needs Increased medical specialisation
United Kingdom	PHC needs Nursing specialisation Population needing care
USA	Populations with unmet needs Physician shortage Enhancement of hospital services
Western Pacific Region	Shortage of health professionals, especially doctors Urgent needs for PHC

Training Programme was instituted to prepare nurses to face an acute physician shortage (WHO, 2005). Approaches to address the unmet needs of a specific population in an urban or rural area will differ as there is more flexibility to engage in longer term planning.

An excess of doctors does not necessarily ensure that services exist to meet all health care needs. However, bringing clarity when identifying the health care needs for a specific population does present an opportunity for health planners to decide who may be best suited to meet these needs, and provides APNs an opportunity to make the case that they are capable of providing services previously undertaken exclusively by physicians. Nurses, physicians and other health professionals working together have the ability to provide complementary services to all populations, especially those who are under-served.

Vignettes 3.1 to 3.5 present illustrations from different countries on how role development has occurred at a practical level in different settings. The vignettes give a sense of the ways advanced nursing is emerging internationally. Illustrations describe improved efficiency in an intensive care unit which is the outcome of the presence of a liaison NP; the diversity of services provided by an NP in a home setting; a situation where the first point of contact for clients is with nurse specialists in a nurse-managed clinic; the benefits that are experienced when NPs are practising in an emergency department; and the psychiatric liaison services provided by a clinical nurse specialist.

Interfacing with nurses, physicians, organisations and the public

In the process of role and practice development numerous questions arise in connection to the APN in relation to interfacing with other nurses, physicians, organisations and the public. In this section the authors provide questions to consider, description of the factors associated with the topics, and strategies to consider in facilitating a smooth introduction of advanced nursing roles.

Interface with nursing

> Are all nurses capable of advanced practice?
>
> Does role expansion for nurses mean a departure from nursing?
>
> Will new nursing roles give support to the professionalisation of nursing?
>
> Will these new nurses lose the 'real' focus of nursing?

The fact that APNs take on some tasks traditionally associated with medicine has raised issues about professional boundaries of nursing. When is a nurse no longer a nurse? Nurses in advanced nursing practice roles express concern about their place in the health system structure, and report poor working relationships with other nurses (Marshall & Luffingham, 1998). In studying structural re-

---

Vignette 3.1　An advanced nursing practice model in intensive care.

The role for the intensive care unit (ICU) Liaison NP was established at Western Hospital, Melbourne, Australia in 1998. Reasons for introducing the role were:

- the complex care requirements for ICU patients
- an acute nursing shortage
- effort to address the issue of preventable admissions and readmissions to ICU
- attempts to reduce delay in identifying and treating medical problems
- optimising use of the limited number of ICU beds available.

To qualify for the role the candidate must have a minimum of 5 years of postgraduate experience. The NP manages new patient referrals during acute phases of instability. This includes initiating laboratory tests, diagnostics and medications, documentation of patient diagnosis, problems and associated observations, direct referral to ICU physician consultants and the ability to initiate discussions regarding advance directives. Ongoing patient management includes preparation for appropriate discharge to the hospital ward, contact with the ward to assure continuity of care, acting as a resource for ward medical staff regarding specific medications, and finally assessment and evaluation of all patients discharged from ICU to the hospital ward. Key responsibilities included in this role are comprehensive patient assessment, grief counselling for family members, consultations with medical staff and initiation of advance directives. Internal evaluation of the role has identified the following outcomes:

- an increase in ICU discharges
- a decrease in preventable readmissions that has led to an increase in ICU bed availability.

Collaborative efforts and regularly scheduled meetings with stakeholders; protocol driven guidelines; and support from key executive staff overcame concerns related to extended practice for nurses and dismissed the perception that this nurse acts as a 'doctor substitute'. With these successes it is expected the hospital will continue to fund the model.

(Green, 2003)

---

arrangement of tasks between nurses and physicians in the Netherlands, Roodbol (2005) found that even though physicians believed that the NP presence had a positive effect on the social identity of nurses in general, nurses as a whole did not share this view and were not prepared to accept the NPs as part of their professional group. Fear that this new type of nurse would consider other nurses to be inferior may have contributed to this perception. This study found that NPs feel conflict about their role expectations. On the one hand the NP is expected to be a nurse; on the other hand expectations of the role associate the nurse more closely with the medical culture.

In the process of introducing APN roles, key informants (personal communication) report that obstacles arise more frequently from nurse than from

---

Vignette 3.2 A nurse practitioner providing home care.

Delivery of care in the home setting fully utilises the assessment skills of the NP while providing professional autonomy. In this vignette home care is provided in association with the Veterans Administration health care system that serves men and women who have completed two years of United States military service with an honourable discharge. The identified patient population is usually older persons who are preparing for end of life. The home care programme works closely with hospital palliative care and community hospice programmes. The physician medical director provides collaboration and medical backup. The hospital cardiology department also provides consultation as needed.

A caseload consists of 33–35 patients with the frequency of home visits determined by the NP, who also assesses the health care needs of the patients. Care is provided in homes, apartments, assisted living facilities and even residential boats. The PHC service includes assessment of health status, ordering and interpretation of diagnostic studies, assisting with the adjustment to new or more appropriate medications, and possible performance of an in home ECG. The NP has the authority to follow and monitor anticoagulation therapy, access bladder scanners for urinary problems, maintain indwelling and suprapubic catheters, as well as provide wound and ostomy care.

Challenges include identifying standard of care for this population and their families while providing and anticipating management plans in the home environment. In providing this type of care the NP is a guest in the patient's home environment; therefore, understanding patient capabilities as well as ability to follow instructions is essential.

(B. Anderson, personal communication)

---

physician colleagues. Gooden & Jackson (2004) point out that few studies have actually been conducted to measure registered nurse (RN) acceptance of these roles. In studying attitudes of RNs toward nurse practitioners, results indicate that RNs believed APNs were knowledgeable, competent health care providers and the generalist nurses were comfortable working with them. However, it seemed the RNs perceived a lack of respect on the part of APNs for the role of the RN in providing patient care. Studies by Bryan (1998) and Roodbol (2005) agree with this finding. The implication is that respectful behaviour among nurses functioning in various capacities is important in providing a team approach for care.

Collegial respect and encouragement

Is collegial respect enough?

Why are nurses reluctant to assist each other?

What concerns make nurses view APN development as a threat?

Vignette 3.3   The nurse specialist as case manager in a nurse-managed clinic.

The first point of contact for HIV/AIDS ambulatory care in Hong Kong is through a nurse-managed clinic. Nurse specialists (NS) provide case management and coordination of services in collaboration with physicians. Clinic services are coordinated with inpatient hospital care under the medical direction of a physician while functioning under the auspices of the Hospital Authority. Individuals concerned with HIV/AIDS approach the nurses when they first seek services. If the nursing assessment reveals an urgent need for hospitalisation a referral is made immediately to the physician in charge. For those requiring less urgent management a history of illness, assessment, blood screening and counselling is conducted with follow-up review of diagnostic blood work two weeks after the initial assessment. Case management and appropriate referral is based on the autonomous judgment of the nurse specialist. Emphasis is placed on assessment of both psychological and physical needs with services extended to partners, spouses and children of clients. The nurse specialist is also the key coordinator of a multidisciplinary care team consisting of a medical social worker, dietitian, psychologist, community nurses and physicians. As team leader this nurse coordinates weekly psychosocial hospital rounds with the entire team in order to provide comprehensive and coordinated hospital, clinic and home care. Department of Health nurses are invited to participate in the team. In addition, the NS facilitates collaboration with the Hong Kong AIDS Foundation, AIDS Concerns and Society of AIDS. These NGOs accept referrals for appropriate services that include transportation, home care and routine follow-up. The nurse-managed clinic provides cost-effective timely care for HIV/AIDS patients based on case management and autonomous decisions of an advanced practice nurse specialist.

(M. Schober, site visit)

Nurses attending a workshop on advanced practice nursing in a location where APN roles were not established commented that they worried about how to gain recognition for this role from other staff, nurses and doctors. These nurses and nursing leaders also sought advice on how to motivate nurses to accept the increased level of responsibility and accountability that comes with practice at an advanced level (Queen Elizabeth Hospital, 2003). At times this fear is justified as often nurses are asked to undertake and accept responsibility for roles in which they have had little or no preparation.

In the United States, schools and colleges of nursing were slow to accept and educate for the APN role. Some nursing leaders opposing the role perceived it as 'selling out nursing' and judged it as an attempt to become a 'junior doctor'. Similar sentiments emerged in the introduction of APNs in the United Kingdom (key informants, personal communication).

A further constraint is that nurses seeking clinical and professional advancement often face heavy work schedules, long work hours and associated fatigue. Options to arrange time off to undertake educational activities and to prepare for a new role are sometimes scarce or restricted. Often there is insufficient

---

Vignette 3.4   Emergency nurse practitioners.

A project sponsored by the Department of Human Services, Victoria began in 2004 in the Melbourne metropolitan area to provide support for the development of NP services in Emergency Divisions (EMDs). The strategy of introducing NPs into EMDs aimed to provide quality and timely care to individuals that could be effectively cared for by qualified nurses. Based on the international success of the NP role, nine hospital-based EMDs collaborated to develop a model of care, a scope of practice and evidence based clinical practice guidelines. Nurses could manage patients presenting at the EMD independently or collaboratively with senior medical staff. In addition, the EMDs joined forces to provide educational opportunities and a support network for NP candidates. This was accompanied by a strong professional and community advocacy to promote, introduce and establish the EMD-NP role.

In assessing outcomes, the project teams in the nine hospitals used similar evaluation strategies and pooled their data to strengthen the value of the results. Findings clearly demonstrated the benefit of the NP service in terms of efficiency and quality of care. In addition to service provision, this unique approach provided the support nurses needed to submit applications for endorsement as an NP in Victoria.

(D. Crellin, personal communication)

Vignette 3.5   Psychiatric liaison clinical nurse specialist.

As a Certified Nurse Specialist (CNS) in Japan this nurse was employed to support nurses and raise the quality of nursing in a municipal hospital in Yokohama in 1995. The CNS programme was new and few nurses knew about the role. In order to promote better understanding of this role visits were made to hospital wards and joint meetings were held with nurses, physicians, clerical employees, psychologists and psychiatrists to provide information and answer questions about the expectations of the role. Periodic discussions were held with the Director and Assistant Director of Nursing to clarify the purpose, activities, effectiveness and CNS issues. This resulted in support from a wide range of nursing administrators. Two years following the introduction of the psychiatric liaison CNS, an oncology CNS was added to the hospital staff.

As a psychiatric liaison the CNS provides case management and consultation on conditions such as adjustment disorders, depression, anxiety, sleep disturbance and delirium. The case management approach includes interviewing and assessing the patient's mental condition and utilises techniques to decrease the person's anxiety. Additionally, in this role, the nurse provides information on the mental health status of the patient's family and informs the physician as necessary. Another responsibility is to be available to support staff nurses who exhibit work-related stress. Clinical management by the CNS includes assessment and recommendations related to pharmacotherapy in consultation with the psychiatrist and pharmacists. The position of the psychiatrist nurse liaison promotes collaboration and team medical management.

(Source: Key Informant, personal communication)

flexibility in the system to allow for study time when holding a paid position, especially when the new role has still to be clearly defined and fully funded. Success in completing educational programmes, whether full- or part-time, is a daunting task when the role is poorly accepted and the environment is unsupportive.

Strategies for promoting positive nursing interface

Nursing supervisors, nursing managers and nurses in various capacities are often responsible for the administration and implementation of services related to the APN. The following recommendations can promote a more harmonious interface of advanced nursing practice with nursing managers and nurses in other nursing roles.

Strategies for interfacing with nursing:

(1) Ensure there is a clear understanding of the role and scope of practice expected of the APN within the specific practice setting.
(2) Make available an explanation of the concept of advanced nursing practice.
(3) Assess nurses' attitudes to identify areas of concern that need to be addressed and consider how best to alleviate areas of anxiety and apprehension.
(4) Facilitate interaction between nurses and APNs to enhance understanding of respective roles, e.g. joint participation in workshops, conferences, and meetings that include management decisions related to both roles.

Interface with medicine

> Why do nurses need these new skills?
>
> Why is there a move to introduce new nursing roles when nurses are needed at the bedside to care for patient populations?
>
> Are APNs mini-doctors, substitute GPs or physician extenders trying to take over the physician role?
>
> Does collaboration and teamwork among doctors and APNs positively influence outcomes in service delivery?

Nurses routinely make judgements and management decisions. This is not a new phenomenon. In certain situations it is possible that competent NPs and APNs could provide a better or equivalent service compared to physicians. Studies have demonstrated that clinical decisions and management provided by advanced nurses compare favourably with those of medical practitioners in terms of quality, safety and accuracy. Reports and analyses demonstrate that these nursing services support high levels of patient satisfaction and quality care. Additional research has highlighted outcomes such as decreased waiting time, improved utilisation of medical and nursing staff, as well as enhanced use and benefit of nursing skills (Buchan & Calman, 2004; Lentz *et al.*, 2004; Horrocks *et al.*, 2002; Mundinger *et al.*, 2000).

The experience of the authors indicates that often physicians are the initial champions of advanced nursing practice, while nursing colleagues desert the novice APN, or fail to facilitate expansion or exploration of education venues and practice sites. A key physician who envisions how the role can complement and enhance overall provision of health care services can be a highly effective advocate (key informants, personal communication). Commenting on working as a physician with NPs in Australia, Gunn (1998) describes positive experiences in palliative care, substance abuse units, sexual health clinics, correctional and Aboriginal health centres. The statement is made that 'greater involvement of nurse practitioners and other non-medical health professionals can only improve our working conditions, benefit our patients and increase our job satisfaction' (p. 2). However, Gunn believes that NPs will only be needed and useful in areas where the medical profession fails to adequately provide services, thus reinforcing the idea that the solution lies in increasing the presence of physicians rather than that of the APN. Drummond and Bingley (2003) comment that the comparison between physicians and APNs is easy for health professionals and the public to comprehend, but tends to promote an adversarial relationship between these groups of professionals.

Over time, the American Medical Association has presented numerous arguments in attempts to defeat support for NPs and APNs. Reasons mentioned include that the APN poses a threat to physicians' income and the power they have over decisions made within health care facilities. The struggle over these issues continues to the present time (key informants, personal communication). In Australia the Australian Medical Association alleged that the introduction of 'nurse practitioners would dumb down' the country's health care system and that 'the addition of these new roles would provide inferior "health care"' (Australia's Independent Voice of Nursing, 2005, p. 1). McGee and Castledine (2003) offer the opinion that opposition by medicine has been less of an issue in the United Kingdom while noting that the conflicts in the interface of medicine and nursing overshadows 'the potential for conflict between advanced practice and other health professions' such as pharmacists, physiotherapists and dieticians (p. 229). The implication is that the interface of all professionals providing health care needs to be considered with the introduction of advanced nursing.

Despite positive descriptions and analysis supportive of advanced practice services, medical dominance as well as control of medicine over health care is cited by key informants (personal communication) as one of the main obstacles that negatively affects implementation of advanced nursing roles. In settings where there are few or no physicians this issue arises infrequently. In environments based on fee-for-service, where financial income is threatened and where there is a surplus of doctors, the addition of APNs to the workforce is not welcomed by medicine. An argument put forth is that as advanced practice educational requirements are less than that of a physician this translates into a lowering of the standards of health care provision (key informants, personal communication). In comparing physician to APN education the question arises: Are there established standards for health professional education that guarantees quality care?

Collaboration

Advanced practice nurses are first and foremost nurses with advanced capability and competence. Where there is a view that achieving quality is an important focus of health care, advanced nursing practice enhances service delivery. This does not mean that APNs are 'substitute doctors' or 'mini docs' but that they have the potential to provide comprehensive nursing care that overlaps minimally with skills and competencies traditionally associated with medicine. It is unimaginable that there is a population in any city or country in the world that would not benefit by the wide-ranging services associated with advanced nursing practice. However, in an environment where there is an excess of physicians and status is threatened by the presence of advanced nursing practice, the ability to support new nursing roles will be extremely challenging. Collaborative strategies can be a way to diffuse conflict arising when adding APNs to the health care workforce.

Evidence from a study conducted under the auspices of the Department of Family Medicine at the University of Ottawa, Canada (2001) supports positive outcomes as a benefit arising from collaboration between physicians and NPs. This research project evaluated structured collaboration. The study findings suggest that collaboration is a learned relationship. A framework that includes a common language for collaborative decision-making is part of the interventional process. Data from this study demonstrate that a structured process does make a difference in how family physician practitioners and NPs behave in organising their work. Findings also indicate that increased understanding of one another's roles and greater confidence in NP competence sustains improved collaboration.

Gidlow and Ellis (2003) cite collaboration as the 'key to success' (p. 161) in promoting advanced nursing roles within a health care team. The authors further suggest that the role boundary shift in doctor–patient and nurse–patient patterns arising from the introduction of APNs could be resolved by creating collaborative affiliations that maintain stability. The resulting teamwork is seen as bringing together the skills and talents of both professions for better care outcomes.

In an editorial for a medical journal, Zwarenstein and Reeves (2000) provide limited evidence suggesting that poor collaboration between physicians and nurses in general leads to poor patient outcomes. Hanson and Spross (2005) document that failure of professionals to communicate can contribute to stress and inefficient service delivery. All this suggests that collaboration can make a positive contribution among health professionals to improve health care but further study is needed to evaluate whether collaborative models of practice have cost-effective benefits and can significantly improve patient outcomes (Schober & McKay, 2004; University of Ottawa, 2001).

Strategies for promoting positive medicine interface

(1) Provide a clear definition of the scope of practice and purpose of the advanced nursing practice roles.

(2) Target key stakeholders such as senior medical officers and medical directors early in the developmental and implementation phases to allow them to contribute to agreement on competencies, develop practice guidelines or protocols, and take part in teaching and precepting of students. These contributions can ease the introduction and promotion of new nursing roles and services.

(3) Inform other professionals and the public regarding the services an APN will be educated to provide.

(4) Establish credible educational programmes to promote role acceptance.

(5) Schedule collaborative meetings, conferences and workshops with physicians to discuss case management and other issues related to the role interface, and take this opportunity to highlight the benefit of advanced nursing practice.

Interface with organisational structures

> Why should nurses seek advanced practice when there is a nursing shortage and nursing skills are needed in the wards of the hospitals?
>
> Advancement of nursing will attract more interest in nursing adding to growth in the profession: is this true?
>
> How will the organisations provide human and financial resources to support the advancement of nursing?

Integrating APNs into the health care workforce is likely to have the effect of changing the type of care provided and location of the service that is available. When considering the option of including APN services, those responsible for decision-making and implementation need to consider the skills and services that these nurses will offer and how these services connect with the organisational structure. Advanced practice nurses should be capable of promoting the benefits of their contributions to health care, and health service administrators should be able to back them by providing an appropriate organisational environment. Without organisational and community support, it may prove difficult to cultivate the job related opportunities and expansions of services that APNs provide.

Where spiralling and rising labour costs are driving health reform, administrators increasingly have to decide what types of health care providers will be cost-effective and provide quality services. The APN will have to demonstrate that a different kind of nursing service will contribute in both of these ways. A clear description of how quality care is defined and can be improved with new nursing roles will strengthen a proposal for a varied and new addition to the workforce. It is important that APNs appreciate factors in the larger health care environment that influence health care. Active participation by nursing in human resource planning and decision-making through providing viable and realistic workforce options is essential (Nevidjon & Knudtson, 2005).

Strategies for interfacing with organisational structures

(1) Build a consensus around role definition, scope of practice, and the settings where APNs will be present.
(2) Involve key stakeholders in discussions on the benefits of APN practice to the organisation's services.
(3) Become involved in organisational workforce planning and skill mix decision making.
(4) Provide outcome studies on patient satisfaction and cost effectiveness.
(5) Be prepared to discuss standards, education needs, options for acquiring necessary education, and regulatory issues.
(6) Establish a framework for strategic planning including follow-up and evaluation of APN services and outcomes.
(7) Provide a plan of options for funding and resourcing for establishing posts, education and continuing professional development.

Interface with the public

Do health care consumers prefer to see the doctor?

Will there be interest in APNs in settings where people are accustomed to going to hospitals for care by physicians and believe it is their right to see a physician?

Will quality of care be inferior when provided by nurses?

Will private patients pay fees to see a nurse?

As discussed earlier, there is evidence that where care has been provided by APNs the public is satisfied with care, and the care is equivalent to that of physicians in specified situations (Buchan & Calman, 2004; Gardner *et al.*, 2004; Horrocks, 2002; Kinnersley, 2000; Lentz *et al.*, 2004). The authors found no evidence to support statements that APNs provide inferior care, or in any way endanger public health.

In the developmental phases in the United States, patients most often openly accepted NPs, while in contrast the roles were questioned by both nursing and medicine (key informants, personal communication). Even though studies have demonstrated patient satisfaction when seen by APNs, it is important that the public is informed of what services can be provided by a nurse in this role. In addressing the issue of promoting the NP role to the public, Buppert (2004) writes that even though evidence demonstrates the benefits, not everyone has experienced care from an APN. For instance, healthy persons or those who rarely use health care services, as well as those who have a long standing relationship with one physician and have no wish to see another provider, are examples of populations possibly unaware of APN services.

In many countries the physician has been the only available option for health care and this has promoted the belief that the physician is the only valid, autonomous health professional. A view exists that where there is an excess of physicians, advanced nursing services are not needed and would be competing with already available care (key informants, personal communication). Conversely, it appears that the provision of complementary and collaborative care provided by APNs is an asset in health care settings (Kinnersley, 2000; Lambing *et al.*, 2004; Lin *et al.*, 2004; Tijhuis *et al.*, 2002). However, careful consideration will need to be given as to how to assure the public as to the safety and quality of these services, as well as to provide information on what APNs can do for them. Professional organisations are just beginning to understand this point and the need for more effective strategies, and the use of a variety of communication methods to describe and disseminate information describing APN services (Buppert, 2004).

Public reluctance and caution in using APN services is understandable when they are unfamiliar with them and lack adequate information about them. However, reports from APNs with experience in this area suggest that after exposure and familiarity with this type of health care provider, users often become the strongest advocates of APN services. Word of mouth communication from patients receiving services on the quality of care, attention to individual concerns provided by the APN, and timeliness in service provision provides a very strong message of the benefits of access to advanced nursing practice.

Strategies for interfacing with the public

(1) Make available specific descriptions of the kind of services APNs will provide.
(2) Identify how APNs collaborate with physicians, other health care professionals and their relationship to the health care facilities.
(3) If there are limitations to APN services, provide clear information about what it is and how to access this service elsewhere, e.g. if the APN does not have the authorisation to prescribe or dispense medicines, how the patient will access drugs.
(4) Use as many methods of public information as possible to introduce APN services e.g. campaigns, articles in publications read by the general public, news media reports, patient advocates.
(5) Organise health talks given by APNs, and raise visibility in the community by offering health screening in settings such as shopping malls, local celebrations or festivals, and consider increasing APN participation in patient associations.

Vignette 3.6 Practising in the absence of legislative or regulatory frameworks.

The United States provides an example of how APN practice initiatives were introduced only to be followed by years of state legal and regulatory battles to develop legitimate authority for APNs. These disputes did not affect all APN roles. Clinical nurse specialists, who were prepared within schools of nursing and employed by hospitals or medical groups, were viewed to be more closely aligned to nursing, and thus less likely to be considered as competition for medical practitioners. The divisive split both with nursing and medicine was with the NPs who strived to practise to the full capacity of their expertise and knowledge level, which included aspects of autonomous assessment, diagnosing and case management. Conflict among the APN fields of NP, CNS, Nurse Midwife and Nurse Anaesthetist contributed to a lack of professional cohesiveness. Even today, there are continuing efforts to secure a legitimate place in the health care arena, obtain satisfactory reimbursement, and resolve regulatory issues.

(Towers, 2005; Key Informants, personal communication)

---

(6) Ensure that APNs participate in community advisory and health policy boards.
(7) Designate and train spokespersons and those responsible for developing communication strategies.

Vignettes 3.6 to 3.10 illustrate approaches and related processes in introducing advanced nursing practice into a country's workforce. Illustrations describe four decades of one country's continuous efforts and achievements, specialisation and career pathway development in another, a university-based master's level clinical education initiative, an NP setting up independent practice, and uneven yet persistent advanced nursing development in another country.

Socialisation: role support

Hixon (2000) writes that socialisation within advanced nursing practice can be viewed as 'three interlinked dimensions: professional socialisation, organisational socialisation, and role socialisation' (p. 46) with the development of 'self' as central to blending all aspects in an effort toward strengthening individual APN identity. Even though Hixon's observations are exploratory in nature, information provided by key informants (personal communication) is consistent with this view. It appears that the emphasis on role acquisition takes place both during the student period and in the transition into a new position when the role is actually implemented in the workplace.

Breaking new ground and being the first individual to provide advanced nursing services can be a solitary experience. Acceptance can be conditional until

---

Vignette 3.7   Simultaneously credentialing for a practice setting and creation of an APN clinical career pathway.

Specialisation in Ireland originated in 1980 with the development of a framework for clinical nurses in 1998. The National Council for the Professional Development of Nursing and Midwifery has the authority to accredit the Advanced Nurse/ Midwife Practitioners (ANP/AMPs). The process for establishing an advanced practice service consists of two parts. Firstly, the service applies to have the job description and site approved for an ANP post. Secondly, the nurse recruited by the service provider seeks to become accredited for that post. A progressive career pathway exists which leads from generalist to specialist, and finally advanced practice. A 24-month masters degree is a required qualification for accreditation as an ANP/AMP.

The clinical career pathway is based on levels of educational preparation, responsibility and level of autonomy. Pay scales are linked to levels of responsibility. The career pathway was created to help experienced nurses grow in their expertise and to encourage them to remain in the clinical field. Policy makers, nurses, unions and service needs were all involved in these developments.

The ANP role is created to meet a specific service need. Once there is a clearly identified need, a job description is agreed and the site is prepared for accreditation, application is made for approval of the ANP or AMP post by the National Council.

(Key Informant, personal communication)

---

that point when the practitioner demonstrates clinical competence and confidence expected of that role. Professional colleagues, health care consumers, and managers, although enthusiastic, may be unable to provide the professional support a new APN requires. Lack of support from other nurses and physicians can be demoralising, especially when there is uncertainty as to the legitimacy of the nurse carrying out tasks or functions that appear associated with medical practice rather than the traditional view of the scope of nursing practice. Professional support at numerous levels appears to strengthen confidence of the individual APN, but evidence as to what kind of support is successful is speculative.

The lag that exists between introducing advanced practice services and arriving at title recognition, scope of practice definition, having access to credentialed educational programmes and finalising appropriate sound professional standards can be lengthy, leaving the new APNs to find their way with no firm frame of reference to guide them. This common phenomenon contributes to a sense of separation and insecurity for pioneer nurses who are doing something that has never been done before. The Queensland Nursing Council (2000) recommends that organisations have definite transitional support strategies to assist nurses entering or returning to the workforce. These strategies serve to facilitate effective application of knowledge and skills while the nurses gain confidence in their practice and practice settings.

Vignette 3.8   An academically-driven advanced nursing practice initiative.

An important feature of Swiss nursing is the presence of a clinical career option that includes nurse specialist-like positions for graduates from post-basic clinical nursing degree programmes. These programmes laid the foundation for the introduction of advanced nursing roles at a later date.

In 2000, the Institute of Nursing Science (INS) at the University of Basel launched the masters in advanced nursing practice with a clear clinical focus. Prior to this, and unlike other advanced university nursing programmes in German and French-speaking countries in Europe, the INS programmes had had a clinical focus, thus placing them in a good position to provide APN education.

Several factors influenced the INS initiative: (1) The need was identified by a number of Swiss nurses and physicians familiar with the Anglo-Saxon models of nursing education and clinical collaboration, and who spent a decade preparing to launch the INS; (2) Findings of a survey of 100 leaders from nursing and other professions that there was a need to invest in more clinically-oriented graduate studies; (3) The return of nurses from study abroad with a clear vision of what could be achieved in advanced clinical roles along with continuing contact with universities in the United States and Europe which helped to strengthen the resolve to move in this direction; (4) The creation of special divisions of clinical nursing science at university hospitals in German-speaking Switzerland that identified one of their goals to be the support of advanced nursing practice. This will be further strengthened by a plan to link these divisions with the INS and form a Swiss Nursing Science Network; (5) A conference held in Switzerland in 2003 to disseminate information on the concept of advanced nursing practice, and numerous lectures and publications.

Another achievement is that INS has secured the guarantee that only nurses will be appointed to the Chair of the Nursing Science Department. This contrasts with some German universities where the unavailability of nurses with the required academic qualifications has resulted in chairs filled by non-nurses leading to a neglect of the core business of nursing.

(Key Informant, personal communication)

Strategies to support new APNs

(1)   Assess individual needs of the APN to develop a suitable plan and strategies to allow the APN to gain confidence in to practice and the application of newly acquired knowledge and skills.

(2)   Set up formal or informal interest groups for new graduates:
   (a)   Providing opportunities to exchange experiences and develop problem solving techniques
   (b)   Communicating options to resolve regulatory, authoritative and institutional obstacles.

Vignette 3.9   Setting up autonomous APN practice.

This vignette provides an example of introducing autonomous APN services in an environment where there had been no previous experience with independent practice. Before embarking on setting up an independent practice in the United States, the NP thoroughly investigated regulations and business practices pertinent to NP practice in order to remain within parameters of state regulations and good business practice. Wide consultation was done with professional nursing associations and legal counsel. In order to establish the format for a profitable fiscal practice, the NP acquired sound knowledge of business practices and followed the necessary steps to establish contacts with physicians willing to work in a consultant capacity. At one point the state medical association challenged the legality of an NP being able to practise independently. Due to the thorough preparatory work that provided a solid legal foundation for independent NP practice that was consistent with state regulations, the NP successfully defended the right to practise independently. The case was further strengthened by success in establishing collaborative relationships with physician colleagues.

(Key Informant, personal communication)

---

(3) Provide educational support through setting up a continuing programme of professional development for graduates:
 (a) Updating skills workshops and conferences
 (b) Enhancing leadership and scholarly expertise
 (c) Clinical evidence-based research practice updates to maintain currency of practice
 (d) Access to publications and information technology.

(4) Identify a mentor who can function as a professional and personal advocate.

(5) Designate funding and resources to support attendance at meetings, conferences and workshops.

Ethical dimensions of the advanced nursing practice role

Are there the distinctive features of ethical decision-making as associated with advanced nursing practice?

The issue of moral and ethical decision-making is basic to all nursing practice. Nurses as well as other professionals in all areas of health care consistently come across moral and ethical dilemmas. However, the APN is in a key position for taking on a more decisive role in managing and creating ethically sound health care settings.

Vignette 3.10   Enthusiastic but uneven advanced nursing practice development.

The idea of having advanced nursing practice has been considered in Macau for over 30 years. In the mid 1970s experienced registered nurses who had received APN training were working in the Government hospital. Nursing professionals and nursing education institutions, under the supervision of the Macau government, first introduced an 18 month APN specialty programme (e.g. mother's health and obstetrics) in 1985. The content of the programme was based on the Portuguese experience, and was taught in that language. In 1992, a diploma programme now taught in Chinese was introduced with courses in gynaecology and obstetrics, paediatrics and community health. Following an examination nurses who had completed the programme adopted the APN role with the title of Nurse Specialist. In 1999 an interruption in programme development occurred and only those specialist nurses who had had the APN qualifications were able to seek promotion. However, such a career move led to only an administrative role thus resulting in the loss of nurse specialists. In the past three years, an APN concept similar to the ICN definition was imported from Hong Kong. Even though the nurse specialist role almost ceased to exist in 2001, privatisation, demands for high quality health care and inspired nursing professionals has led the Macau Government and interested health care professionals to begin to plan to introduce advanced nursing practice education at the masters level. Since the handover of Macau to China nurses appear to have more possibilities to influence health care policy. However, there are continued threats to APN development such as the authority and high ratio of the doctors to nurses [1:1.1], inadequate governmental support and a nurse population not necessarily interested in promotion or change. Regardless of the lack of APN role clarity and confusion regarding education, titles and functions, there is a plan by nurse educators and regulators to restart an advanced practice programme in Macau.

(Key Informant, personal communication)

An in-depth discussion of ethical decision-making is not within the scope of this chapter; rather this section will highlight the level of ethical decision-making that is evident in advanced nursing practice. (The reader is referred to the ICN publication *Ethics in Nursing Practice: a Guide to Ethical Decision Making* [Fry & Johnstone, 2004] for a comprehensive and practical text on this topic specifically written for the global nursing community.)

An ethical or moral predicament occurs when responsibilities require, or appear to require that a person adopt two (or more) alternative actions, yet the person cannot carry out all the necessary actions. Conflict occurs when varying demands and choices exist, all of which can be equally objectionable (Hamric & Reigle, 2005). For example, an APN may oppose mandatory HIV/AIDS screening within occupational health settings because it goes against concepts of client autonomy and confidentiality, while also recognising that lack of adequate identification limits access to appropriate therapies and could result in transmission of the virus to other employees.

The ability of APNs to take part in ethical decisions evolves from their clinical expertise and the development of collaborative skills. Skills including ethical decision-making in practice situations along with clinical expertise and leadership enable nurses in advanced practice to critically analyse and manage the decision-making process.

Advanced practice with associated independent responsibilities for patients has altered the interface between nurses and physicians when facing an ethical situation. Conflicts based on differing professional views with dual professional accountability occur more commonly in advanced nursing practice and are usually connected to conflicts over patient care management (Fry & Johnstone, 2004) as is illustrated by the situation that follows.

> *A nurse practitioner in a general practice clinic saw a 45-year-old woman who was concerned about superficial bruising and swelling affecting her ankle that had been noticeable for three days. She lived in another country and was visiting her mother for three weeks. Previously she had been a patient in this clinic and trusted the doctor she had consulted on prior occasions. On a visit two years before, it had been noted that her blood pressure was slightly elevated, she was beginning to notice perimenopausal symptoms, and was obese. The NP, after taking a history and performing an examination determined that the bruise and swelling was secondary to an injury received four days prior to this visit and probably associated with trauma when the woman stepped on the edge of a concrete step and fell. Her management plan was treatment for the ankle injury, observation of response to treatment, and a return visit in one week for evaluation. In a spirit of collaboration, the NP reviewed the case with the practising physician in the clinic. The physician discounted the patient's concern about the ankle, ordered a full blood chemistry profile as well as a pelvic ultrasound while reprimanding the patient for gaining weight. Prescriptions for hypertension and anxiety were written for the woman even though her blood pressure on this visit was within normal range and she had not exhibited any evidence of anxiety. Although not totally irrelevant to the case the NP felt the recommendations were excessive and failed to address the main reason for the woman's visit. The patient voiced concerns about the cost and time involved in following the physician's recommendations.*

Should the NP point out her disagreement with the management plan to the physician?

Analysis

What is the significance of the values involved?
The NP wants to provide cost-effective, competent care appropriate for the problem without compromising the total health status of the woman. The physician has a sound reputation, explains in detail the rationale for the plan but does not seem to value the findings and opinion of the NP. To the NP the physician's management plan appears to be excessive, costly and inap-

propriate for this visit. However, to take action means the NP would have to confront the physician about this disagreement.

What is the significance of the conflict to the involved parties?
Nurses, including those in the capacity of APN, find that not to agree with the physician is so unpleasant that everything is done to avoid confrontation. The authority of the physician is usually accepted without question. In this way the NP–physician relationship remains intact, and the physician views the NP as obedient and collaborative. The NP could take the patient aside and provide her additional advice but this would undermine her credibility and the patient's trust in the physician.

What should be done?
While it is important to uphold collegial relationships the NP, given her increased level of knowledge and accountability has an additional responsibility to facilitate reasonable, cost-effective and credible care. This means that the task of discussing the situation and related concerns openly with the physician cannot be ethically avoided.

(Ethical decision-making format adapted from Fry & Johnstone, 2004)

Even though this situation occurs in an ambulatory care setting, it demonstrates that a critical aspect in the nature of the nurse/physician interaction when managing the care of any patient is the ability to discuss and value each other's opinions. While the situation depicted is not life-threatening, an inability to discuss disagreements over therapeutic management or end-of-life decisions frankly may in the end place patients in jeopardy if professionals follow dissimilar plans.

Conclusion

Information provided by key informants, experiences of the authors and examples of success provided in the literature have provided examples of what works in the process of APN role and practice development. Factors that appear to promote successful initiatives for advanced nursing practice include:

- Strong education programmes for the generalist nurse that provides a sound basis for the nurse to pursue advanced nursing roles
- Flexible and realistic educational options that not only prepare competent APNs but offer possibilities to bridge the gaps of educational preparation when countries are in a transitional phase for programme development
- An identified need for the APN and associated clinical career pathways
- Available role models and active mentorship
- Access to appropriate expert consulting that is a continuous and sustained contact over time
- Presence of nursing leadership in ministries of health and health departments
- An active visible presence of APNs

- The ability of organisations to perform when including advanced nursing in the workforce.

Pivotal decisions on how nursing practice will advance are dependent on positions taken by influential persons who may have diverse levels of understanding as to the place APNs should occupy in health care systems. Initiatives and schemes begin for different reasons and proceed in random ways. Advanced practice nurses appear to strengthen and enhance health services, but the process of implementation is likely to be uneven and challenging. Factors to consider when introducing advanced nursing practice, as well as examples and illustrations of strategies that have met with some success, have been provided. It is hoped that they will help those embarking on this journey to identify issues and possible solutions as they arise on the road towards having vibrant, competent APN services.

References

Ang, B.C. (2002). *The quest for nursing excellence.* Editorial. *Singapore Medical Journal,* **43**(10): 493.

Australia's Independent Voice of Nursing. (May 2005). Nurses slam AMA's 'dumbing down' slur. *Nursing Review.* Canberra: RCNA. www.nursingreview.com.au

Bryan, S. (1998). School nurses' perception of their interactions with nurse practitioners. *Journal of School Nursing,* **14**(5), 17–23.

Buchan, J., Calman, L. (2004). *Skill mix and policy change in the health work force: Nurses in advanced roles.* OECD Health Working Papers, No. 17. DELSA/ELSA/WD/HEA (2004) 8.

Buchan, J., Dal Poz, M.R. (2002). Skill mix in the health care workforce: Reviewing the evidence. *Bulletin of World Health Organization,* **80**(7), 575–580.

Buppert, C. (2004). *Nurse practitioner's business practice and legal guide,* 2nd Edition. Sudbury, MA: Jones and Bartlett Publishers.

Canadian Nurse Practitioner Initiative. (2005). *Overview of the Canadian Nurse Practitioner Initiative.* Retrieved August 26, 2005 from www.cnpi.ca

Community Tool Box. (Undated). *SWOT analysis: Strengths, weaknesses, opportunities, and threats.* Retrieved 22 December, 2005 from http://ctb.ku.edu/tools/en/section_1049.htm

Drummond, A., Bingley, M. (2003). Nurse practitioners in the emergency department: A discussion paper. *Canadian Journal of Emergency Medicine,* **5**(4), 276–280.

Fry, S.T., Johnstone, M-J. (2004). *Ethics in nursing practice: a guide to ethical decision making.* Oxford: Blackwell Publishing.

Gardner, G., Carryer, J., Dunn, S., Gardner, A. (2004). *Nurse Practitioner Standards Project: Report to Australian Nursing Council.* Australian Nursing Council: Author.

Gidlow, A., Ellis, B. (2003). Advanced nursing practice and the interface with medicine in the UK, in P. McGee, G. Castledine (Eds), 2nd Edition, *Advanced Nursing Practice,* pp. 157–183. Oxford: Blackwell Publishing.

Gooden, J.M., Jackson, E. (2004). Attitudes of registered nurses toward nurse practitioners. *Journal of the American Academy of Nurse Practitioners,* **16**(8), 360–363.

Green, A. (2003). *ICU Liaison Nurse Practitioner Model.* Presentation for Nursing Symposium 2003 'Advanced Practice Nursing: Perspectives and Challenges', Central Nursing Division, Queen Elizabeth Hospital, Hong Kong. Feb. 14, 2003.

Gunn, A. (1998). Nurse practitioners are a benefit not a threat. DRS (Doctors' Reform Society) column of *Australian Doctor,* 13 March 1998.

Hamric, A.B., Reigle, J. (2005). Ethical decision-making, in A.B. Hamric, J.A. Spross, C.M. Hanson (Eds) *Advanced practice nursing: an integrative approach*, pp. 379–412. St. Louis, Mo: Elsevier Saunders.

Hanson, C., Spross, J.A. (2005). Clinical and professional leadership. In A.B. Hamric, J.A. Spross, C.M. Hanson (Eds) *Advanced practice nursing: an integrative approach*, pp. 301–339, St. Louis, Mo: Elsevier Saunders.

Heifetz, M. (1993). *Leading change, overcoming chaos: A seven stage process for making change succeed in your organization.* Newberg, Oregon: Threshold Institute.

Hixon, M.E. (2000). Professional development: socialization in advanced practice nursing. In J.V. Hickey, R.M. Ouimette, S.L. Venegoni (Eds) *Advanced practice nursing: changing roles and clinical applications*, 2nd Edition, pp. 46–65. Baltimore: Lippincott Williams & Wilkins.

Horrocks, S., Anderson, E., Sailsbury, C. (2002). Systematic review of whether nurse practitioners working in primary care can provide equivalent care to doctors. *British Medical Journal*, **324**, 819–823.

International Council of Nurses. (2005). *Health Policy Package (HPP)*. Geneva: Author.

Kinnersley, P. (2000). Randomised controlled trial of nurse practitioner versus general practitioner care for patients requesting 'same day' consultations in primary. *British Medical Journal*, **320**: 1043–1048.

Lambing, A., Adams, D.L.C., Fox, D.H., Divine, G. (2004). Nurse practitioners' and physicians' care activities and clinical outcomes with an inpatient geriatric population. *Journal of the American Academy of Nurse Practitioners*, **16**(8), 343–352.

Lentz, E.R., Mundinger, M.O., Kane, R.L., Hopkins, S.C., Lin, S.X. (2004). Primary care outcomes by nurse practitioners in patients treated by nurse practitioners or physicians: Two-year follow-up. *Medical Care Research and Review*, **61**(3), 332–351.

Lin, S.X., Gebbie, K.M., Fullilove, R.E., Arons, R.R. (2004). Do nurse practitioners make a difference in provision of health counselling in hospital outpatient departments? *Journal of the American Academy of Nurse Practitioners*, **16**(10), 462–466.

Marshall, Z., Luffingham, N. (1998). Does the specialist nurse enhance or deskill the general nurse? *British Journal of Nursing*, **7**(11), 658–661.

McGee, P., Castledine, G. (2003). Future directions in advanced nursing practice in the UK. In P. McGee, G. Castledine (Eds), 2nd Edition. *Advanced Nursing Practice*, pp. 225–237. Oxford: Blackwell Publishing.

Ministry of Health, New Zealand. (2002). *Nurse practitioners in New Zealand.* Wellington: Author.

Mundinger, M.O., Kane, R.L., Lentz, E.R., Totten, A.M., Tsai, W.Y., Cleary, P.D., Friedewald, W.T., Siu, A.L., Shelanski, M.L. (2000). Primary care outcomes in patients treated by nurse practitioners or physicians: a randomized trial. *Journal of the American Medical Association*, **283**(1), 59–68.

Nevidjon, B.M., Knudtson, M.D. (2005). Strengthening advanced nursing practice in organizational structures and cultures. In A.B. Hamric, J.A. Spross, C.M. Hanson (Eds) *Advanced practice nursing: An integrative approach*, 3rd Edition, pp. 845–874. St. Louis, Mo: Elsevier Saunders.

Nursing Council of New Zealand. (2002). *The nurse practitioner: responding to health needs in New Zealand*, 3rd Edition. Wellington: Author.

Overseas Development Administration. (1995). *Guidance note on how to do stakeholder analysis of aid projects and programmes.* Retrieved 22 December, 2005 from http://www.euforic.org/gb/stake1.htm

Professional Regulation Commission, Board of Nursing, Manila. (2002). *Nursing Specialty Certification Program* BON Res. No. 14 S. 1999 and *Guidelines for Implementation* BON Res. No. 118 – S 2002. Manila: Author.

Queen Elizabeth Hospital. (2003). Preworkshop survey results of nurses attending a workshop on advanced practice nursing. Hong Kong: Unpublished.

Queensland Nursing Council. (2000). *Transition support processes.* Position statement. Brisbane: Author.

Roodbol, P. (2005). *Willing o'-the-wisps, stumbling runs, toll roads and song lines: study into the structural rearrangement of tasks between nurses and physicians.* Summary of doctoral thesis presented to authors. Unpublished.

Schober, M., Mackay, N. (2004). *Collaborative practice in the 21st Century.* Monograph 13, Geneva: ICN Author.

Tijhuis, G.J., Zwinderman, A.H., Hazes, J.M., Van Den Hout, W.B. Breedveld, F.C., Vliet Vlieland, T.P. (2002). A randomised comparison of care provided by a clinical nurse specialist, and inpatient team, and day patient team in rheumatoid arthritis. *Arthritis Rheumatology,* **47**(5), 525–531.

University of Ottawa, Family Medicine Department. (2001). *Nurse practitioner/family physician structured collaborative practice.* Final Research Report to Health Transition Fund Secretariat, Health Canada. Retrieved August 9, 2005 from http://www.icn-apnetwork.org

World Health Organization. (2005). *WHO supports integrative management of childhood illness and advanced practice nurse training in Timor-Leste.* Public Information and Events, 3 (2). Retrieved June 21, 2005 from w3.whosea.org/LinkFiles/Public_Information_&_Events_vol3-2_timor-leste.pdf

Zwarenstein, M., Reeves, S. (2000). What's so good about collaboration? We need more evidence and less rhetoric. *British Medical Journal,* **320**(7241), 1022–1023.

Chapter 4
Regulation

Introduction

In 1986 when the International Council of Nurses (ICN) examined structures and standards regulating nursing education and practice around the globe, it found nursing to be:

> *. . . ill-defined and diverse; educational requirements and legal definitions of nursing generally inadequate for the complexity and expansion of the nursing role as it is emerging in response to health care needs (ICN, 1986, p. 43).*

Today, a similar state of confusion exists for advanced nursing practice even in countries with a long history in this field of nursing. Advanced nursing practice is struggling to be recognised, to establish appropriate practice standards, to decide on what kind of education is required, and to have its scope of practice legitimised and applied in health systems. This situation was summed up by key informants (personal communication) from one country in this way:

> *The 'good news' has been the flexibility of the role. The 'bad news' is the resulting crazy quilt or hodgepodge of role descriptions, titles, scopes of practice related to the specifics of the extended role skill set and educational and registration requirements.*

All these issues appear to be related in part to the absence of professional regulation, or the nature of the regulatory framework in place. To achieve consistency as well as to endure and evolve, advanced nursing practice needs a regulatory/legislative framework.

This chapter will explore the key elements required to create a regulatory/ legislative framework that meets ICN standards for regulation, and suggest a model that permits advanced nursing practice to evolve as a distinct and legitimate part of the health delivery system in a country.

The regulatory/legislative framework

The ICN definition of professional regulation is broad, acknowledging the growing and dynamic scope of professional regulation, and thus making it able to encompass and adapt to changes and role progression. For ICN regulation includes:

> *. . . all legitimate and appropriate means – governmental, professional and private – whereby order, consistency, identity and control are brought to a profession (Styles & Affara, 1997).*

In general it is possible to distinguish three layers or tiers in professional regulatory/legislative frameworks for nursing (Affara & Styles, 1992). These layers are illustrated in Table 4.1.

(1) At the highest layer, the statute (law, decree or ordinance) is the supreme statutory instrument. As a minimum it will give legal recognition to advanced nursing practice through definition of the advanced practice nurse (APN) and title protection. Often the law will designate an implementing body (Nursing Board, Council, Committee), and delineate its powers and functions. Laws are more durable and difficult to alter. While specifications embedded in the law will be better protected, they are less open to change. Usually, the higher a regulatory element is placed in the legislative framework, the more rigorous is the process for approval.

(2) At the next layer, rules and regulations (or bylaws) further amplify the law. Rules and regulations undergo less scrutiny as normally they do not have to be approved by the law-making body of the country. Often ministerial

approval is sufficient to give rules and regulations the power of law. Processes, procedures and requirements for credentialing of the APN, standard setting, accreditation of educational programmes, and professional discipline may be found at this level. For example, the law may simply state that its purpose is to provide for the licensure, education and discipline of APNs, and then specifies functions and powers (e.g. making regulations, implementation and enforcement of the law) delegated to a designated body. This entity will be responsible for setting standards, and developing as well as implementing the processes and procedures needed to operationalise the law.

(3) The third layer deals with implementation and interpretation matters, issues that arise out of application and enforcement of the law. These are usually the responsibility of the designated regulatory body, if one has been named in the law. Interpretative powers will allow the regulatory body to elaborate and give guidance to licensees and others on the law and regulations. For example, while the law and/or regulations may specify the level of educational qualification required, the regulatory body can use its interpretative powers to define minimum curriculum content and produce guidelines for the conduct of educational programmes to meet its criteria. The scope of practice may be defined in regulations or bylaws, but guidelines addressing specific aspects of the scope in greater detail may be issued in response to new practice situations or emerging trends (Affara & Styles, 1992).

Table 4.1 Layers in regulatory/legislative framework. (Source: Adapted from Affara & Styles, 1992.)

Layer	Purpose	Authority
I. Statute/Law/ Ordinance/Decree	To provide statutory authority for the profession	Legislature/President/ Head of Government/ Minister
II. Rules and Regulations (bylaws, secondary legislation)	To further expand the law. Identify in greater detail how the legislation is to be enacted	Minister/Nursing Council or other delegated body (e.g. Professional Association)
III. Implementation and Interpretation	To apply the law and rules and regulations; to communicate the content law/rules/regulations through further elaboration e.g. guidelines, codes of practice	Nursing Council or other delegated body (e.g. Professional Association)

Vignette 4.1 Practice restricted by law.

In the early 1970s a small Caribbean country established an NP programme to prepare nurses to work in health centres to reduce the need for continuous physician presence at health centres. As NPs were to assume responsibilities such as prescribing drugs and treatments until now restricted to physicians, nursing and medicine collaborated closely to introduce the role. Initially the plan was to pass legislation before NPs began to implement the role so that NPs were legally covered to practice in an expanded role, including having prescription privileges. For various reasons this was not done and NPs were introduced into the country's health system. However, what was forgotten was that, by law, pharmacists could dispense only those prescriptions signed by a physician. As a result prescriptions NPs signed were illegal, and therefore were not dispensed by pharmacists.

(Cumper, 1986)

The type of regulatory/legislative framework occurring in a country can fundamentally affect the nature and range of professional practice. Just as it can impede and restrict the evolution of advanced nursing practice, it can be instrumental in facilitating and promoting growth and orderly development of the role. For an example of how it can restrict practice see Vignette 4.1.

Factors influencing the regulatory/legislative systems

It is important to become cognisant of and understand the impact of factors in the context in which regulation occurs as these are likely to influence the structure of the system. The policies, practices and mechanisms adopted, including how well professional regulation is able to cope with new or changing circumstances, and the degree of professional control afforded by the system, can be affected by numerous external factors as demonstrated in Table 4.2.

Credentialing advanced nursing practice

In 1997 ICN took note of the considerable growth and interest in the credentialing of nurses for specialist or advanced practice roles, and the accreditation of institutions and programmes offering nursing education or services. Credentialing is considered by ICN as part of the broader concept of professional regulation. It is defined as:

processes used to designate that an individual, programme, institution or product have met established standards set by an agent (governmental or nongovernmental) recognised as qualified to carry out this task. The standards may be minimal and mandatory or above the minimum and voluntary. Licensure, registration, accreditation, approval, certification, recognition or endorsement may be used to describe different credentialing processes . . . Credentials may be periodically renewed as a means of assuring continued quality and they may be withdrawn when standards of competence or behaviour are no longer met (Styles & Affara, 1997, p. 44).

Thus, credentialing is a central function of a regulatory system. A credential denotes a level of quality and achievement that can be expected in terms of

Table 4.2 Factors likely to influence the regulatory/legislative framework.

Factors	Aspects to note
Type and stability of the political system in the country	Is there strong central government control or are powers devolved to regions? Is it a federal system? Are there frequent changes in the ruling party and/or Ministers?
Legal and regulatory traditions of the country	Are professions regulated solely through a government controlled process? Is professional self-regulation a common practice? How strictly are laws related to professional regulation enforced? What are the stages and processes for enactment of laws and regulations? What types of credentialing mechanisms are commonly used?
International trends and influences in regulation	What is the impact of regional and international trade agreements? Is there a significant level of emigration or influx of health professionals into the country? What influence do international credentialing agencies have in the health and education sectors?
The degree of specificity or generality sought in the regulatory system	How broadly worded is the primary legislation? At what level is detail to be found in the regulatory/legislative system?
The rapidity of change in educational standards, practice and technologies	How rapidly are new knowledge and technology applied in health and education? At what stage of evolution are the nursing, educational and health systems? How open are they to change and innovations?
The time required, cost and expertise, both financial and human, for enacting and/or revising laws and regulations, and for implementing regulatory systems	How complex is the process for introducing new, or modifying current elements in laws, or other legal instruments and policies? How rapidly do the involved institutions respond? What are the main methods used to advocate legal or policy change? Are they effective? What access is there to expertise and resources for advocacy work?

standards met, competence shown and behaviour exhibited by the credentialed entity, whether it is a nurse, a programme of study, a service provided, or the institution in which education or service programmes are offered. Often a credential carries an exclusive right for the person or the agency to bear a designated title, and to provide specified services (Affara & Styles, 1992).

Mandatory credentialing occurs when the authority is the law. However, there are situations where voluntary credentialing is sought if the credentialed entity (nurse, institution, educational programme) wishes to demonstrate the quality of the service or expertise offered is above that required by statutory regulation (Styles, 1999). Examples include: Korean nurses seeking certification from the American Nurses Credentialing Center (ANCC) demonstrating that they have reached a level of excellence from a reputable credentialing body; the Spanish Nurses Association seeking international recognition through becoming an approved provider of continuing education of ICN's international continuing nursing education credits (Bernal, 2005); or nursing services acquiring a magnet hospital designation accreditation which recognises the excellence of the nursing services (ANCC, 2005).

The authors propose to use the ICN Credentialing Framework, first adopted by the ICN Credentialing Forum in 2001, to examine key issues related to regulating the APN role. The framework, drawn from the definition of credentialing, is useful in exploring how *order*, *consistency*, *identity* and *control* are achieved in regulating APNs and their practice. It assists us to collect data pertinent to a credentialing system. It can be used in a national or international context, applied to a whole system or to a specific category of health worker within a system (ICN, 2004).

Components of the credentialing framework

The eleven components or elements (Table 4.3) forming the framework deal with descriptions of the entity being credentialed, and the structures and processes of credentialing. A description of each component follows with examples of how they have been applied to advanced nursing practice around the world.

The credentialee

The recipient of the credential, the credentialee, is the APN and in some cases the educational or service programme or institution.

As discussed in Chapter 2, deciding what title to confer can be problematic as advanced nursing practice tends to evolve, at least in the initial stages, in the absence of well-developed definitions communicating spheres of responsibility and accountability. ICN takes the position that the name must convey a simple message of who is the APN. It should allow us to distinguish the APN from other nurse categories (Styles & Affara, 1997). When little discrimination is made in defining advanced practice roles in relation to other extended or specialised

Table 4.3 Components of the ICN credentialing framework.

Credentialee
  Target:
    Health care provider
    Educational programmes institutions
    Service programmes/institutions

Credentialer
  Government
  Professional organisations
  Non-professional non-governmental
    agency/agencies
  Other

Mechanism
  Authorisation
  Certification
  Endorsement
  Licensure
  Recognition
  Registration
  Others

Duration
  Awarded for:
    Indefinitely
    For specified period
  Can be revoked/suspended

Purpose
  Practice restriction
  Title restriction
  Definition of scope of practice
  Setting standards for education
  Setting standards practice
  Definition of professional accountability
  Promotion of high quality practice
    and service
  Recognition of distinctive practice
  Provision of information to consumers,
    employers, payers
  Others

Processes
  Verification through:
    Acquiring educational qualifications
    Tests/examinations
    Practice requirements
    Self-assessment
    Portfolio development
    Peer review
    Interview
    Transcript review
    References
    Professional discipline
    Others

Powers
  Practice protection
  Title protection
  Accreditation of educational/service
    programmes/institutions
  Approval of scope of practice
    statements/job description/posts
  Others

Funding/costs
  Sources of funding:
    Initial/renewal of credential
    Sitting examinations
    Programme/institution accreditation
    Credential checking
    Government funding
    Consultation services
    Sales of materials
    Other
  Costs:
    Administrative
    Development of verification tools
    Communication, information,
      advocacy

Standards/competencies
  Entry into APN education programmes
  Entry into APN practice
  Accredited of programmes/institutions
  Parties involved in setting standards/
    competencies:
    Government
    Regulatory authority
    Nursing profession
    Other professions
    Public
    Others

Effectiveness
  Collecting information about and
    tracking credentialees
  Research
    Relevance, reliability of
      credentialing processes
    Impact on client outcomes

Mutual Recognition Agreements
  Within same country
  Other countries

Vignette 4.2   Practising without title protection.

To increase access to health services, a country with a good health infrastructure began to prepare nurses in a variety of advanced practice roles. This occurred in the absence of national agreement on role definition, title and standards for education and practice. As a result each health authority and even individual health facilities interpreted advanced nursing practice to suit their particular need, often choosing a title that described the post rather than the role. The result was a proliferation of titles, role confusion, variability in standards and uncertainty as to how to develop this role further across the health system. One nurse working in this context expressed how she felt about the lack of official recognition of the role she was carrying out in this manner: 'I use the skills I have to make a difference for patients. But those patients have no way of checking that I am what I say I am. They take me on trust! Of course they also measure me by the outcomes achieved.'

(Key Informant, personal communication)

---

roles and levels of practice, role definition tends to proceed in a disorderly and reactive manner, and titles proliferate (Castledine, 2003; Gardner *et al.*, 2004; key informants, personal communication).

As the major reason for title protection is to safeguard the public from unqualified practitioners who have neither the education nor the competencies implied by the title (see Vignette 4.2), regulatory bodies take this aspect of credentialing seriously, and may even go as far as trademarking the title, as was done by the Nursing Council of New Zealand (NCNZ) prior to obtaining legal title protection (key informant, personal communication).

Credentialing mechanisms

Credentialing mechanisms refer to processes used to regulate the APN. They include the conferral of academic diplomas or degrees, accreditation, approval, authorisation, certification, endorsement, licensure, recognition and registration.

Credentialing the advanced practice nurse

Regulatory mechanisms differ, and the method selected is often linked to a country's regulatory traditions and resources, as well as judgement of what level of regulation is required to authorise a nurse working beyond the legally recognised scope of practice for a registered nurse (RN). Thus each jurisdiction will opt to develop 'criteria and processes to meet the expectations and requirements of legislation, health departments, and the public' (Gardner *et al.*, 2004, p. 69). This adds to the variability in the way the role is defined, credentialed and put into practice.

In deciding on the type of regulatory mechanism required certain factors are taken into consideration. They include:

- Perceived potential and level of risk, and likely severity of harm to the consumer
- Depth of specialised and advanced knowledge required
- Skills and abilities needed for practice
- Degree of autonomy allowed by the role
- Breadth of scope of practice (National Council of State Boards of Nursing [NCSBN], 2002).

A number of mechanisms may be employed for regulating advanced nursing practice, and as has been mentioned previously, the final choice will depend on the character of the regulatory environment (see Table 4.2). The most common mechanisms used are:

- **Licensure** This is the most restrictive form of credentialing and it usually provides for title protection, defines the qualifications, and restricts certain practice rights to nurses holding the licence. It involves the application of validation processes to ensure that the nurse is safe to practise in the specified scope, and has met predetermined standards. While licensure carries with it a high level of accountability and has strong public protection intents, it may stifle the evolution of practice of the generalist nurse who is excluded from providing any of the services specified in the APN scope of practice.
- **Certification** This mechanism enables an individual to demonstrate that certain predetermined standards have been met. It may also confer the use of a certain title such as certified nurse. However, certification in itself does not limit practice to the certified nurse. Regulatory bodies may use certification obtained from professional associations in place of their own certification during a licensure process.
- **Registration** In its purest sense registration means that an individual's name has been entered into an official register for persons who possess specific qualifications. The register is maintained by the regulatory or another official governmental body, and usually provides title protection. There is no inquiry or validation of the competence of the nurse. Some jurisdictions may require an APN to be registered and have a licence or practice certificate. A licence or practice certificate is usually the aspect that needs to be renewed periodically if the nurse wishes to continue practising.
- **Recognition** Sometimes known as designation, recognition consists of an authorised body such as a nursing council granting permission for nurses with specified credentials to represent themselves as nurse practitioners or clinical nurse specialists or any other specified title without undertaking verification of competence. While recognition does not give exclusive practice rights or title use, it does serve to provide information that a person has special knowledge, skills and expertise in a field of nursing (NCSBN, 1993; Porcher, 2003).

As there is no international consensus on the definition of these terms, caution is advised in interpreting the form of credentialing said to be in place. It is necessary to go beyond the name given to the actual credentialing mechanism to verify exactly what is entailed in becoming credentialed, and the rights and protections it carries. Readers are referred to the Glossary for definitions of the terms proposed by ICN for international use.

Since the early 1990s, the need to hold a second licence as opposed to certification with title protection as the necessary level of legal authority for advanced nursing practice has been debated in the United States. Given the level of complexity, specialisation, and independent decision-making required of today's APN, a second licence is proposed (NCSBN, 2002; Porcher, 2003). Others argue that the RN licence is the foundation for advanced nursing practice, at least for the CNS, and a second licence is an example of 'over-regulation' although it is recognised that 'optional regulations should specifically speak to practice in the medical domain and should not be construed to be requirements for CNS practice in nursing's autonomous domain authorised by the RN license' (National Association of Clinical Nurse Specialists [NACNS], 2003).

The American Association of Colleges of Nursing (AACN, 1998) takes the position that credentialing should be limited to assuring that specified educational qualifications are attained and that competence to practise is affirmed through a national certification process that validates and standardises qualifications and practice competencies nationally.

Other countries report that they regulate APNs through registration. However, as licensure and registration are often used interchangeably, registration may be interpreted differently from one jurisdiction to another. In many cases registration requires passing through some type of validation procedure, and will confer title protection. It may also bestow exclusive practice privileges, and is therefore nearer in form to licensure than to the pure form of registration. For instance, in Ontario Canada, nurses are registered as 'extended class registered nurse'. They are RNs who 'have obtained advanced education and passed the Extended Class examination'. These RNs become RN(EC) and have 'an expanded scope of practice in the areas of assessment, diagnosis, ordering of tests and prescribing treatments, and health promotion' (College of Nursing of Ontario [CNO], 2004).

Singapore has recently amended the Nurses and Midwives Bill to create a register for APNs. The Bill provides for title protection, qualifications, education, standards and mandatory continuing education. While it defines a scope of practice, it is not clear whether certain aspects of advanced nursing practice will be restricted to persons on the register (Singapore Ministry of Health, 2005).

Regulatory bodies, mostly in Australia and New Zealand, have chosen what is called authorisation (New South Wales) or endorsement (Victoria and New Zealand). These mechanisms may define the field of practice, scope and conditions of practice in the expanded scope. These specifications vary among jurisdictions, even within the same nation (Gardner *et al.*, 2004; Lewis & Smolenski, 2000; NCNZ, 2002; Nurses Registration Board of New South Wales, [NRB], 2003; Nurses Board of Victoria [NBV], 2004; Professional Regulation Commission Board of Nursing, Philippines [PRC], 2002; key informants, personal communication). For instance, New South Wales ties authorisation to use of the NP title, and certain privileges such as prescribing medications from a formulary, ordering diagnostic tests and making limited referrals so long as these conform to guidelines approved by the Director General of the Health Department (NRB, 2003). This latter proviso highlights a contentious issue that has emerged in other countries. Guidelines or protocols specific to APN practice, or requirements for some form of physician supervision are seen to carry the risk of being overly restrictive and inhibiting innovative responses to new and changing situations that are inevitably encountered during APN practice. Also, they may become another way for others, especially physicians, to exert control over professional practice (Gardner *et al.*, 2004).

In Ireland, the National Council for the Professional Development of Nursing and Midwifery (2004) links the credential to a job description and the site where the APN will practise, both of which need approval by the Council's accreditation committee. By 2005, 30 advanced nursing credentials had been approved (ICN Credentialing Forum, 2005). A person can hold the credential so long as he or she is working in an approved post in same specialty. The credentialing process is called accreditation, although this term is usually applied to educational or service programmes, institutions or facilities.

Certification may be used on its own, or part of number of licensing requirements. Many United States nursing boards require proof of certification from a recognised certification agency. In the United States certification has many players as certifying bodies for the different nursing specialties that have emerged. Lewis and Smolenski (2000) note that it has become a complex issue as it 'can be used for entry into practice, validation of competence, recognition of excellence, and/or regulation' (p. 75). One result, as Hanson (2005) points out, is 'a multiplicity of certification configurations of advanced nursing practice certification' (p. 792). In an effort to improve the quality and enhance the uniformity of certification processes, national organisations such as the American Board of Nursing Specialties or the National Commission for Certifying Agencies recognise voluntary certification programmes that meet defined standards (Bernreuter, 1999).

One issue surfacing in countries where professional organisations have strong traditions in standard setting especially in the specialty nursing area, is whether credentialing of advanced nursing practice should be left to the professional association, a model adopted by many other professions. This point has been under discussion in New Zealand where the New Zealand Nurses Organisation (NZNO) conducted voluntary certification programmes for nurses practising at an advanced level until the 2003 Health Practitioner Competence Assurance Act extended the power of regulatory authorities to set scopes of practice and assess competence throughout the practitioner's professional life. Nurse practitioner regulation then became part of the regulatory body mandate. Currently, while NPs are credentialed by the Nursing Council, the NZNO has retained voluntary

certification for a category named *nurse clinician* (NZNO, undated; key informant, personal communication).

In Japan, advanced nursing practice credentialing is solely a professional responsibility. The Japanese Nurses Association (JNA) and other professional associations conduct certification programmes (ICN Credentialing Forum, 2004).
Korea has adopted a joint approach where the credentialing authority is the
Ministry of Health and Welfare, but certification is managed by the Korean
Nursing Association or the Credentialing Centre for Nursing Education (Kim,
2003). However, in Thailand the Nursing Council is the certifying agent and the
credentialing authority (key informant, personal communication).

As previously mentioned, the degree of authority and type of limitations
placed on privileges (e.g. prescribing, ordering laboratory tests, referring, admitting to hospital) granted varies across jurisdictions. This is very evident in the
discussion on prescriptive authority in Chapter 2, which also points out that
approaches to prescriptive authority are mirrored in the wider debate on the
advanced nursing practice role, and reflects the confusion that surrounds role
evolution, definition and regulation around the world.

Accrediting educational institutions and programmes

Credentialing mechanisms may target APN educational programmes. The
mechanism most commonly used is accreditation, although in some countries
the term approval or recognition may be used. ICN defines accreditation as:

> *a process of review and approval by which an institution, programme or specific
> service is granted a time-limited recognition of having met certain established
> standards beyond those that are minimally acceptable (ICN, 1997, p. 41,
> update 2004).*

Accredited educational programmes communicate to the profession, policy
makers, employers and citizens that advanced nursing practice has established
educational standards and through an accreditation system continually reviews,
monitors and enforces them. This serves as a guarantee that graduates from
accredited programmes have met certain specified criteria. Also, well-developed
accreditation systems play a part in ensuring that advanced nursing practice
education remains abreast with developments in the fields of health and nursing sciences, practice developments and educational methodologies. While
the benefits of having accredited programmes may be evident, problems
especially when the concept is new or unfamiliar need to be acknowledged. They
include:

- Application and preparatory costs related to fees, document preparation, faculty development required to meet accreditation standards, personnel time
  for preparing for accreditation, and expenses if remedial action is necessary.
- The accreditation processes themselves may be excessively demanding and
  burdensome, especially in situations when it needs to be sought from more

than one authority e.g. professional regulatory body and the agency accrediting higher education.

- It may engender feelings of resentment and threat in a faculty unprepared or insufficiently involved in the accreditation process.
- Inconsistent application of standards or criteria may undermine the credibility of the system (ICN, 1997).

As most advanced nursing practice programmes tend to be in the higher education sector, accreditation by the agency responsible for that sector may already be compulsory. However, in some jurisdictions professional regulators require that advanced nursing practice education is obtained from programmes approved or accredited by them (NRB, 2002; key informants, personal communication). Other parties also consulted and involved in setting standards for education are organisations such the National Organization of Nurse Practitioner Faculties (NONPF) and various APN professional organisations in the United States. Both types of group have been in the forefront in promoting quality education. They have done so through promoting standards and guidelines, and identifying criteria for programme evaluation, and now are collaborating with other countries such as Canada and the United Kingdom in NP development (Pulcini & Wagner, 2004). In the United Kingdom, where the advanced nursing practice role has evolved in the absence of regulation, the Royal College of Nursing (RCN) now offers voluntary accreditation for educational programmes. It is interesting to note that prior to creating the accreditation unit, the RCN used a franchise model to validate and maintain some consistency in RCN-NP programmes offered by other institutions (RCN, 2002, revised 2005).

In 1997, ICN identified a number of broad policy objectives to underpin educational institutions and programme accreditation. They continue to be relevant as a basis for developing the more specific standards for advanced nursing education, programme management and institutional requirements. The ICN policy objectives can be used by authorities to establish standards for education and set up accreditation processes for nursing programmes and institutions offering the programmes. The policy objectives are broadly stated and sensitive to the contextual factors that need to be considered. They are:

- Accreditation of schools of nursing is for the purpose of protecting the public by ensuring that nursing educational programmes prepare graduates that are able to meet the standards for competent, ethical and appropriate professional practice as defined in that country.
- The curriculum and teaching/learning experiences promote competencies required to practise competently, ethically and appropriately. Assessment methods relate directly to these competencies. Periodic reviews occur to assure the continuing relevance of competencies, curriculum and teaching/learning methodologies.
- The educational programme identifies and prepares for the full range of competencies that the graduate with that particular qualification will be required

to demonstrate for practice. Preparation includes the capacity to take on all responsibilities connected with that professional role as defined in that country.

- Educational programmes encourage the full development of the student's potential in nursing and as a citizen through liberal, social, scientific and technical education.
- Nursing research is valued and reinforced.
- Key stakeholders – the government, citizens, employers, educational institutions, the nursing profession, other health professions and others – have an interest in the preparation of nurses. Appropriate participation by these groups in accreditation processes is desirable e.g. on committees dealing with accreditation of schools of nursing, on the school board, on student selection committees.
- The reason for the participation of interested parties in the accreditation processes is made explicit and is appropriate. Policy setting and processes used are not dominated beyond their legitimate interest by the government or its appointed participants or any one group within and outside the profession. Multiple and competing interests are recognised as may happen when management and the accreditation of schools are vested within the same authority.
- Regulation is sufficient to accomplish the purpose i.e. there is neither too much or too little.
- Processes focus largely on accrediting the programme, administrative and educational and assessment processes, faculty and facilities (for theoretical and clinical teaching/learning).
- Broad guidance is provided on required subject areas, faculty specifications and learning resource requirements rather than over-detailed prescription of procedures and curriculum content. Diversity of approach is encouraged and seen as a legitimate way to reach educational outcomes.
- Accreditation processes are established in such a way that there is coordination among the different parties involved (e.g. statutory body regulating the profession, agencies with responsibility for oversight of educational programmes in a country e.g. ministry of education, educational institutions) and different levels (regional, national and local). Processes avoid duplication and overlapping of function and clearly define areas of responsibility.
- While jurisdictions may adopt temporary measures to accommodate existing conditions, broad and uniform development of the profession mandate that standards of education match the increasing rigour of health care requirements and are relevant to the local needs. As the globalisation movement takes greater hold the need for international credentials and, therefore, the development of universally acceptable standards becomes more important.
- Standards and procedures are relevant and full information is provided regarding criteria and processes e.g. for admission to programmes, assessment

and disciplinary procedures. Objective measurement and review are used, reasons for decisions reached are given and there is opportunity to appeal decisions.

- Nursing education fits within the dominant educational pattern in the country and occurs in the same setting, at the approximate level, and with similar autonomy as for other professions. If it is customary for physicians and other health professionals to serve on nursing education boards, it is equally fitting for nurses to serve on the boards of other health professionals. Nursing has opportunities equal to that of other health professions to participate in the process of regulatory and educational policy and decision-making in areas that relate to nursing and health (ICN, 1997).

Standards for education and accreditation grow out of these policy objectives. Figure 4.1 suggests areas where standards should be developed to suit a country's specific needs and possibilities. The reader is also advised to consult the resource section at the end of the book where examples of programme accreditation standards and processes are given.

Philosophy and goals of education

Organisation and administration of the institution and programme

- Structure, organisational policies and relationships
- Director
- Faculty
- Personnel policies
- Budget
- Documentation

Curriculum

- Content
- Implementation of curriculum
- Curriculum evaluation

Students

- Selection
- Polices
- Rights and responsibilities

Resources and facilities

- Faculty
- Classrooms/laboratories
- Clinical learning sites
- Library, electronic and other teaching/learning resources
- Other school facilities
- Support services

Figure 4.1   Areas for setting accreditation standards. (Source: ICN, 1997.)

Credentialer

Who conducts or administers the regulatory processes? The agent of credentialing may be the government or non-governmental agencies such as specialty boards or professional associations offering voluntary certifying or accreditation programmes (Henderson, 1999; ICN Credentialing Forum, 2004; RCN, 2002 revised 2005). When there is statutory (mandatory) credentialing, the responsible agent is usually named in the related legislative instrument.

There is often collaboration between statutory regulatory bodies and voluntary agencies in advanced nursing practice credentialing. For instance, a nursing board charged with licensing APNs may recognise certification conferred by APN and NP professional organisations or other certifying bodies as being valid as a requirement for practice.

Purpose

Purposes of credentialing vary. They range from public protection to ensuring the safety and competence of the credentialed entity. Credentialing may be devised for one or more of the following purposes:

- Protecting the public by keeping unqualified individuals, organisations, and services from the field
- Establishing that requirements for practice have been met
- Defining scope of practice and standards for education and practice
- Establishing professional accountability
- Granting exclusive use of title to a credentialed entity
- Defining rights and privileges
- Promoting high quality practice and service
- Recognising distinctive practice
- Informing employers, payers and consumers about the special attributes and qualities of the APN or services offered so that they can make informed choices (Affara & Styles 1992; Styles, 1999).

It is important that credentialing is relevant and capable of achieving stated purposes. ICN takes the position that the overriding purpose of credentialing is protection of the public by providing them access to safe, competent care. Therefore, to achieve this goal the credentialing system needs to safeguard that:

- Standards of education are appropriate and are subject to regular review for continuing relevance
- Practice standards are pertinent and are evaluated periodically for validity in the face of changing circumstances
- Verification methods used are reliable and relate directly to standards
- Scope of practice remains relevant to responsibilities conferred on APNs (Styles & Affara, 1997).

Powers

Powers refer to the authority given to the credentialing agent to enforce title protection, to restrict the field of service to credentialed individuals, organisations or institutions, to make rules and regulations, and to issue interpretations. While the power of the law is supreme, in models of professional self-regulation depending on the system, varying degrees of power will be conferred on the profession. The greater the power the greater is the freedom given to the profession to decide on standards. In 2005, a joint statement by ICN and the World Health Organization (WHO) reaffirmed that self-regulation should continue to underpin 21st-century regulatory systems for nursing (ICN-WHO, 2005).

Standards

Standards and competencies lie at the heart of a credentialing system as they define the quality of performance required of a credentialed entity. Standards set the level of education and performance for entry into practice and for renewal of credentials (Figure 4.2). Competencies define the level and quality of performance the credentialee is expected to demonstrate as a practising APN. Other standards may exist for educational programmes and institutions offering them. The authors recommend ICN's international principles for standards development as a useful resource when establishing, reviewing or evaluating standards (Appendix 4).

Entry into practice standards

- Current RN registration/license
- Specified educational requirements usually from an accredited programme
- Passing a specified examination or other form of competency assessment e.g. certification, interview, portfolio review
- Specified number of practice hours in a certain time period – may be linked to a specific practice area
- Approved job description or scope statement and/or approved post
- Evidence of indemnity insurance

Renewal of licence standards

- Specified amount of continuing education
- Re-examination (re-certification)
- Specified number of practice hours in a certain time period including proof that it is carried out within authorised scope of practice
- Interviews
- Portfolio up-date
- Random audit
- Evidence of indemnity insurance
- Research achievements, publications, conference and other forms of presentations

Figure 4.2 Examples of standards for entry into practice and renewal of licence. (Source, Key Informants, personal communication.)

Deciding who to involve or consult is an important first step in standards setting. Key informants (personal communication) reported a wide range of groups involved: the profession in general, APNs and relevant specialty groups; educators; nursing and education regulatory authorities; the government (policy- and decision-makers); employers and health services managers; other professions especially physicians and pharmacists; and consumers and patient groups. In New Zealand, the Nursing Council is required to consult with the profession (key informant, personal communication). It does so through the Nurse Practitioner Advisory Committee, which has membership from four key nursing associations. In South Africa, the Nursing Council and professional organisations work with the South African Qualifications Authority, the body responsible for setting general standards for education and training in the country for all tertiary and higher education (key informant, personal communication). In Taiwan the Ministry of Health has set up a national NP Council to oversee a number of working committees, including those involved with standard setting (Chao, 2005).

What emerges from the experiences of key informants (personal communication) is the need to be well aware of the context, to be strategic and to embrace a philosophy of being inclusive when selecting partners and groups to participate in identifying scope, standards and competencies, especially when the role is unfamiliar and contested.

Processes

This component of the credentialing framework refers to the processes or procedures used to validate or verify that standards are met.

Processes for validation of competence to practise are various and may include examination, portfolio review, application desk audit, interview or assessment by an expert panel, as well as practice and continuing education requirements (Hanson, 2005; NBV, 2004; NCNZ, 2002). Figure 4.3 identifies some of the areas countries have included in the portfolio.

As Vignette 4.3 demonstrates, in situations where advanced nursing practice is not well established and nurses have not been able to access the exact qualifications now required, difficulties may occur in obtaining recognition of prior education and experience. This transition period is a delicate process to manage as it requires regulatory bodies to be sensitive when evaluating prior experience, learning and formal qualifications for equivalency.

Term or duration

A credential may be bestowed for life, it may be revoked under certain circumstances, or be valid for a specified period only. In most countries familiar to the authors, the period of validity may vary from one to ten years. Usually, renewal is conditional on having met certain requirements in the preceding period, such as having practised a specified number of hours in the relevant field, or

An organised collection of documents demonstrating education, experience, knowledge, competencies and capabilities in an area of advanced nursing practice, and shows the depth and scope of practice undertaken by the applicant, as well as a capacity to analyse and reflect on practice.

A portfolio may include:

- Evidence of leadership in practice e.g. mentoring, contributions to improving practice
- Evidence of current licence
- Scope of practice statements, job descriptions and supporting evidence that verifies advanced skills, competencies and knowledge in practice
- Curriculum vitae outlining work and educational history
- Educational qualification – verified certificates and transcripts, or full details of educational programmes undertaken when seeking recognition of educational equivalence
- Referees and/or written letters of support/references
- Performance reviews and peer evaluations
- Documents illustrating practice – e.g. case studies; work diary; involvement on initiatives such as policy formulation, clinical guidelines or protocol development in relevant area of practice; educational programmes delivered
- Scholarly activities – research, publications, projects undertaken
- Membership and involvement with a professional organisation
- Evidence of professional indemnity insurance

Figure 4.3 Examples of contents of a portfolio. (Source: NCNZ, 2002: NBV, 2004.)

Vignette 4.3   Difficulties in obtaining recognition of prior education and experience.

An NP candidate with 14 years of experience and holding two graduate diplomas pertinent to the field of practice applied to be endorsed as an NP in a country where advanced nursing practice was in the early stages of evolution. The qualifications were accepted by the university as being equivalent to a masters degree. However, this assessment of the academic qualifications was not accepted by the Nursing Board who required the candidate to undertake full masters degree studies, as well as a course in therapeutic medication management. The nurse decided to discontinue her effort to become an NP.

(Key Informant, personal communication)

---

providing proof of continuing competence and/or continuing education. It may involve taking a re-certification examination as indicated in Figure 4.2. Several key informants (personal communication) have pointed to the fact that, given the newness of regulating APNs in some jurisdictions, initial and renewal credentialing processes are still being tested and modified.

Costs

Credentialing has cost implications for the individual nurse and the credentialing agency. The nurse is expected to pay fees to acquire the initial credential and for subsequent renewal. Costs may include expenses related to preparation for, and a fee to sit, the examination.

Credentialing bodies are likely to incur considerable costs in producing and administering validating instruments and carrying out verification processes, particularly when it involves developing examinations. The estimated cost for developing a new certification examination, including role definition, may be 115 000–130 000 USD, and could take up to two years to develop (D. Paulson, personal communication). In addition, modern credentialing systems require significant financial and human resources to administer the system; maintain databases; communicate, report, and disseminate information; advocacy work; and hire required expertise.

A credentialing system may be well designed, but without sufficient resources for its operations may find it is unable to carry out essential tasks adequately, and may fail to maintain its pertinence and dynamism. This is especially problematic in small countries with fewer APNs. Even in countries with the potential to credential large numbers as in Japan, the JNA is uncertain whether it will be possible to maintain current levels of rigour, effectiveness and efficiency of credentialing when numbers seeking credentials rise (ICN Credentialing Forum, 2004).

A recent consultation in the United Kingdom reported concerns around the costs to APNs of initial registration and re-registration (NMC, 2005). Another aspect is the considerable effort and time invested by individual nurses in preparing or updating portfolios and studying for certification (Gardner *et al.*, 2004; ICN Credentialing Forum, 2004). Key informants (personal communication) also highlighted the cost of education as being a significant impediment, even in the richer countries. Nurses seeking to practise in this role may have considerable social and financial responsibilities. In a country with limited resources such as Sudan, the price tag of 3000 USD per year for undertaking a master's programme is a major obstacle (A. Osman, personal communication). One way to overcome such obstacles is for individual nurses to align their professional development goals to that of the employer.

The perspective of the employer needs to be taken account of with respect to costs. Meeting the credentialing demands of the different groups of health care providers, as well as institutional accrediting standards, can impose significant costs for employers. Certification and accreditation does not come cheap. Processes can be complex and time-consuming for all involved. How do employers and management justify and defray the accompanying cost, juggle the time issues associated with multiple accrediting and credentialing requirements, and yet run an efficient organisation that respects its fiscal limits?

Close consideration of how to create an adequate regulatory system which is also achievable within available resources is important. It may mean limiting credentialing to registering the APN without verification of the competence of the applicant, but ensuring that good role definition, well-defined competencies and adequate educational programmes are available. Aspects dealing with programme and institutional accreditation need to be coordinated with other agencies that may be charged with these responsibilities. For instance, are their standards congruent with those sought by the nursing regulatory body? Is it possible to strengthen their accreditation standards or persuade them to adopt standards proposed by nursing?

Another action would be to look closely at how often the credential needs to be renewed, and the type of requirement asked for renewal. Are they feasible and reasonable? For instance, if the APN must undertake a certain number of hours of approved continuing education, is it available locally, and within the financial means of nurses? Renewal requirements should be congruent with what is available and achievable in a nurse's situation.

Effectiveness

Increasingly credentialers are being asked to produce evidence related to the quality of performance of the regulatory system, and the degree to which credentialing is meeting its stated purposes. Unless evidence exists to confirm that credentialing is operating efficiently and does contribute appreciably to assuring better and safer health services, governments, nurses, employers and others will challenge the need to expend resources for this purpose. Regulators should be interested in exploring whether evidence confirming that credentialing improves health services does indeed exist.

Questions to explore include:

- What is the relationship between credentialing and public protection and quality of services?
- What evidence is there that APNs need to be credentialed?
- Which assurance measures are likely to produce predictable outcomes in credentialing e.g. what type of education, how credible are validation procedures such as examination, portfolio review, interview, and prior approval of scope of practice statements?
- What care outcomes differences, if any, exist between credentialed and uncredentialed nurses caring for similar patient groups?
- What are the cost–benefit outcomes of having credentialed health professionals providing care?
- What kind of documentation and data collection processes are needed to assure competent research in credentialing? (Cary, 2001)

Mutual recognition agreements (MRA)

Mutual recognition acknowledges and recognises that credentials from another jurisdiction meet equivalent standards and have the same rights as the equivalent credential in the host jurisdiction. It is described as a process where:

two or more parties agree to recognise and accept all, or selected aspects of each other's regulatory results because they are harmonised or judged to be equivalent, or because they satisfy other agreed-upon external criteria. Results may include assessment outcomes, qualifications, standards, rules, titles, and quality assurance system standards (Adapted from Trans Atlantic Consumer Dialogue [TACD], 2000).

In our interconnected world, migration and the importation of health personnel to combat shortages is becoming big business. This means that more nurses now desire to practise in venues other than the one in which they were educated and licensed. Additionally, there are more instances where health care services and educational programmes are being delivered across borders in the form of telehealth and e-education services. Mutual recognition is one of the mechanisms used to deal with professional recognition issues arising as a consequence of the free movement of services and persons promoted by globalisation and international/regional trade agreements (Affara, 2004).

Mutual Recognition Agreements (MRA) may exist between sovereign countries, or are in place in nations with multiple jurisdictions, as in Australia, Canada and the United States (Affara, 2004). The Trans Tasman Mutual Recognition Act of 1977 between Australia and New Zealand is an example of an MRA between two countries. The act requires that nurses from the signatory jurisdictions, among other groups, be mutually recognised in all jurisdictions named in the Act. Consequently, Australian and New Zealand regulatory bodies have identified a core role description, core competency standards, and educational standards for NPs (Gardner *et al.*, 2004).

Model for a regulatory system for advanced nursing practice

Based on the concepts described in the ICN Credentialing Framework, a regulatory model is proposed (Table 4.4) that has the following characteristics.

- **In the law** The definition of the advanced practice nurse; title protection; the nature of the body charged to regulate the APN (e.g. composition, appointment, term of office); functions; powers to conduct affairs (e.g. make regulations, interpret, enforce the law, raise revenue); and ways to deal with nurses from other jurisdictions are given the level of protection afforded by the law.
- **In the regulation/bylaws** Elements more sensitive to alterations in practice, knowledge, technology and patterns of health care delivery are dealt with through regulations/bylaws, or through interpretation thus permitting sufficient flexibility to respond to the health system, professional and other societal changes.

As discussed earlier in the chapter, the degree of specificity required and the level at which regulatory elements are placed will vary according to a country's regulatory and legislative traditions, and other factors impinging on the regulatory context. For instance, some jurisdictions protect the title in the law, while others place title protection in regulations. In a wide ranging review of legislat-

Table 4.4 ICN model regulatory system. (Source: Adapted from Affara & Styles, 1992.)

Law	Regulations/Bylaws
Definition of APN	Scope of practice definition

Title Protection	Standards and guidelines
	   Entry into practice
	   Education
	   Practice
	   Assuring continuing competency
	   Professional conduct

Regulatory body
Composition
Powers and functions
Appointment and conditions for office
	Processes/procedures for certain regulatory
	  activities
	Credentialing
	Holding examinations, reviews, interviews
	Accreditation of educational programmes/
	  institutions
	Renewal, suspension, removal,
	  reinstatement of licence
	Hearings/consultations
	Complaint and disciplinary proceedings

Dealing with other jurisdictions	Communication Reporting
Resources for conducting affairs (power to raise revenue)	Data collected about credentialees Evaluating regulatory effectiveness

ive and regulatory frameworks currently available in Canada, and in the few countries with APN regulation (Australia, New Zealand, United States) carried out for the Canadian Nurse Practitioner Initiative, Tarrant (2005) noted inconsistencies among jurisdictions in the following areas:

- The range of regulatory elements included in the available regulatory/legislative instruments (law, rules, and regulations) i.e. what was included from the elements detailed in Tables 4.3 and 4.4
- The level of detail used in regulatory instruments
- The positioning of the regulatory elements i.e. how they were distributed among the levels present in a jurisdiction.

The model suggested gives those countries with no or rudimentary systems of regulation a structure to begin to pursue the regulatory changes or reforms that the profession needs to survive in the 21st century. The ICN/WHO (2005) future perspective envisages '. . . patient safety and public protection continue to be paramount goals'. It sees the '. . . application of global education and practice standards and competencies allows nursing to define more clearly and consistently its role and the services it can offer', and '. . . career and clinical

- Understanding the current system
- Articulating clear and descriptive definitions that make APN responsibility and accountability explicit
- Going beyond initial assessment to ensure continued competence of the APN, and relevance and quality of education
- Creating a system sufficiently responsive to altering health care needs and the expanding capabilities of nurses

Figure 4.4 Regulatory challenges. (Source: Adapted from Styles & Affara, 1997.)

pathways, including frameworks for advanced practice and nursing specialties, benchmarked against international standards'.

Many barriers and complexities still face advanced nursing practice as it searches to establish viable regulatory policies and practices that promote quality advanced practice nursing services as well as support its progressive development. Figure 4.4 identifies some of the multiple and sometimes complex challenges that may be encountered in developing a sound system to regulate advanced nursing practice.

Exploring your regulatory environment

Preparation

You will need sufficient copies of documents such as statutes; rules and regulations supplementing statutes; relevant policy statements; official definitions of the advanced nursing practice, scope of practice; categories recognised, titles used; guidelines; and accounts and reports of current credentialing policies and practices. Remember you may need to consult other areas (see Vignette 4.1), Acts, policies and laws (e.g. in public health, pharmacy, control of medicines, mental health, and labour) that may have provisions regulating nursing practice. You may wish to speak to persons who have passed through the credentialing procedures to understand the system from the user point of view. If you have undertaken the SWOT analysis and stakeholders analysis suggested in Chapter 3, you are likely to find that analysis will be pertinent to this task. You may wish to add to your understanding of context by repeating both activities but this time focusing specifically on the regulatory environment.

Forming an overview of the regulatory/legislative systems

The questions that follow should give you a point of departure. You can use them to explore some of the broader legislative/regulatory issues in the country or jurisdiction.

(1) What is usually included in (a) the law, and (b) the regulations governing professions in your country?

Table 4.5 Stakeholders' role in establishing the regulatory/legislative framework.

	Legislature	Regulatory body	Profession	Public members	Others, specify
Scope of practice protection					
Title protection					
Designating the regulatory body including powers and functions					
Establishing definitions of APN					
Delineating scope of practice					
Setting standards for: Entry into practice Education Practice Continuing competence					
Setting policies and procedures for: Initial/renewal authorisation to practise Accreditation of educational programmes Filing complaints and professional discipline					

(2) Given the circumstances in the country, what do you think needs the protection of the law?

(3) Where do you want to put the emphasis in the system – ensuring APNs are qualified and maintain competence; accrediting educational programmes; or assuring quality of the practice environment? It may be all three, or that the tradition in your country is to focus on one or two of those mentioned, or that resource limitation (financial, availability of expertise) force you to make choices. What do you think is necessary and feasible for the advanced nursing practice role?

(4) In creating a regulatory/legislative framework for advanced nursing practice in your jurisdiction who are (a) likely to be major decision-makers, and (b) whom would you ideally wish to be involved in making decisions about the areas given in Table 4.5? Consider for each of the tasks listed on the left hand side of the table what stakeholders you need or would wish to involve in decision-making: legislators, regulatory body, the profession, and others such as public representatives or other professionals.

Understanding regulatory and legal frameworks for advanced nursing practice

Once you have a broad overview of what is going on in the regulatory environment, it is important that you are familiar with the characteristics of, and processes of, that current practice, or that are likely to be used to regulate advanced nursing practice in the event that regulation is sought. You can use this exercise to build on the information you have already acquired when forming an overview of the regulatory system in place.

We suggest that you use the ICN Credentialing Framework (Table 4.3) and Model Regulatory System (Table 4.4) as checklists to verify what currently exists (structure, policies, processes and practices) for nursing generally, and advanced nursing practice specifically. If you are already credentialing APNs, this exercise can be used to evaluate the system. It can help you identify areas of strength, weakness, gaps and redundancies. Where APNs are not being regulated, but where there is a desire to establish a structure and related policies and practices, you can use the process to scan the current regulatory/legislative environment prior to developing a specific plan for that purpose. If APN regulation does not exist, examining what is happening in health professions regulation in general will help you understand the regulatory climate in your jurisdiction.

Some questions to focus on are:

- Is/are the purpose/s of regulation clearly stated?
- Are all essential definitions included? Are they clearly expressed and complete? What areas need more development?
- Does the regulatory agent have sufficient powers to carry out the stated purpose for regulation? Are there problems with enforcement? What are they?
- What evidence exists that point to satisfaction or dissatisfaction with the performance of credentialees? What do credentialees think of the system – is it fair, does it give good value, and is it responsive to their needs?
- What do other key groups think of the system?
- How many complaints are received, from whom and about what?
- Are there out-dated requirements, policies and procedures?
- Are the features of the system consistent with one another and the stated purposes of regulation?
- Is the system operating with sufficient resources (human and financial) to enable it to operate efficiently, provide appropriate services, and remain relevant?

Advocating for regulatory/legislative change

One of the themes running through the key informants' responses is dissatisfaction with the state of regulation for APNs, or the adequacy of current policies and practices, leading to role confusion, definitional inconsistencies, lack of recognition, and uncertainty in boundaries of practice. Nurses need to be effective advocates for a regulatory framework that is capable of defining, legitimising, maintaining quality and sustaining advanced nursing practice roles.

Advocacy is not new as individuals or groups have always tried to influence people in power (International HIV/AIDS Alliance, 2002). There are many definitions of this word but probably the most useful one for our purpose is: 'an action directed at changing the policies, positions and programmes of any type of institution' (Sharma, R. Undated).

Only two aspects of advocacy action have been selected for further discussion:

(1) Analysing and understanding policies, laws, rules and other related documents.
(2) Planning and applying advocacy strategies.

The reader is invited to refer to the resources section for more information on advocacy work.

Document analysis

Understanding the effects of policies, laws, rules, administrative orders and other instruments that regulate nursing is essential when you are seeking to introduce new regulatory initiatives, or to change current regulatory provisions. It is important to understand what the existing documents are actually saying and to note if possible:

- Who benefits from this legislation or policy?
- Who loses?
- Who supports this law/policy and why?
- Is it being enforced? If yes, by whom, and how? If not, why is this?

In exploring these questions it may help you to judge if the documents are:

(1) Supportive to your goals or needs, or have to be dealt with in a way to reduce the harm they may cause to your plans.

(2) Reality matching what is actually written in the texts. Are the policies, laws, rules and regulations being enforced? If this is not so, it will be important to discover why this has happened as it will be important information to use in making your case, and in proposing change.

Advocacy strategies

One of the factors influencing success in this area is the ability to plan and apply effective advocacy strategies directed at changing the legal and other regulatory provisions affecting APN recognition, practice and education. Some of the tools used to advocate for change are give in Figure 4.5.

There are some basic rules to remember when carrying out advocacy work (ICN, 2005; International HIV/AIDS Alliance, 2002; Sharma, R., undated):

(1) Have a good knowledge of the broader environment. Carry out the environmental scan suggested in Chapter 3. This will help you to understand the formal and informal decision-making process and identity who the deciders are.

(2) Identify the audience you need to address – key decision-makers, and individuals and groups that can influence decision-makers.

(3) Establish relationships and strategic alliances or networks with key players. While creating networks and coalitions takes time and energy as they involve building relationships of trust, establishing such ties is an effective way to add weight to proposals and opinions. Although there may not always be full agreement, if there is respect and a professional approach, the relationship may work. If possible, make sure that the people affected by the issue are involved in defining it, and planning advocacy strategies from the beginning. They will have expert knowledge of the situation, and will add strength and legitimacy to the advocacy work.

(4) Write and publish strategically. That means timing and the place where the information is published and disseminated is important. Take up opportunities to speak to influential groups.

(5) Communicate positions through representation on policy-making committees or boards, lobbying, making submissions, meeting with people in positions of influence. Always consider who the audience will respond to and find credible.

(6) When developing positions, briefings or other advocacy messages be concise about what you want to achieve, why and how. Use positive approaches to strengthen the case by being positive about the good parts found in official documents related to the issue; responding only in those areas where there is something concrete to offer; using language in the way it is understood and employed by decision/policy-makers; and ensuring that written statements are clear and professionally presented.

(6) Prepare well and support the case/proposal/statements with facts and evidence where possible. Refer to Chapter 6 for more information in using research for advocacy purposes.

(7) Offer solutions.

- Analysing and influencing legislation or policies
- Identifying the audiences you need to address
- Developing advocacy messages and choosing an appropriate delivery format:
    - Preparing a briefing note or position paper
    - Lobbying or face-to-face meetings
    - Delivering presentations
    - Using press releases
    - Giving a media interview or press conference

Figure 4.5   Advocacy tools. (Source: International HIV/AIDS Alliance, 2002.)

Conclusion

Legislation and regulation should confer identity, legitimise the role, and grant clear authority to carry out the range of activities pertaining to that role. However, in the international arena the literature and observations from key informants suggest that considerable problems, impediments and differences occur in the way advanced nursing practice is regulated. There is a constellation of issues around:

- Titling (what name and the level of protection)
- Scope of practice particularly in relation to what is included and the level of authority accorded to carry out the scope e.g. autonomous practice or under some form of protocol or supervision
- Educational requirements
- Types and rigour of the credentialing mechanisms used in initial and renewal of credentials
- Methods used for validating competence.

To assist with thinking about and establishing viable regulatory/legislative frameworks, the authors have proposed tools for exploring the regulatory environment, and suggest a model to assist with development of appropriate and adequate regulatory structures, policies and practices.

References

Affara, F.A. (2004). *Understanding mutual recognition agreements*. Geneva: International Council of Nurses.

Affara, F.A., Styles, M.M. (1992). *A nursing regulation guidebook: From principle to power*. Geneva: International Council of Nurses.

American Association of Colleges of Nursing. (1998). *Position statement: Certification and regulation of advanced practice nurses*. Washington: Author. Retrieved 8 August, 2005 from http://www.aacn.nche.edu/Publications/positions/cerreg.htm

American Nurses Credentialing Centre. (2005). *Benefits of becoming a magnet designated facility*. Retrieved 4 July 2005 from http://www.nursingworld.org/ancc/magnet/benes.html

Bernal, M.O. (2005). *Spanish pilot project: Report on the ICN international accreditation system for continued education in nursing*. Paper presented at the ICN 23rd Quadrennial Congress, Taipei, Taiwan. Retrieved 22 July 2005 from http://icn.ch/RegulationConference2005/presentation/OvalleBernal_files/frame.htm

Bernreuter, M. (1999). Accrediting the accreditors in nursing: the American Board of Nursing Specialties. In A. Cary, C. Wharton (Eds) *Quality assurance through credentialing: Volume 2 – Concepts, issues and trends*, pp. 43–48. Washington: American Nurses Credentialing Centre.

Cary, A. (2001). *Outcomes of credentialing: Developing, analysing and implementing evidence*. Presentation given at ICN Regulation Network Meeting at the 22nd ICN Quadrennial Congress.

Castledine, G. (2003). The development of advanced nursing practice in the UK. In McGee, P., Castledine, G. *Advanced nursing practice* (2nd Edition), pp. 8–16. Oxford: Blackwell.

Chao, Y.M.Y. (2005). *Designing nurse practitioner system in Taiwan.* Paper presented at the 23rd ICN Congress, Taipei.

College of Nursing of Ontario. (2004). *Registration extended class: Fact sheet.* Toronto: Author.

Cumper, G. (1986). Neglecting legal status in health planning: Nurse practitioners in Jamaica. *Health Policy and Planning,* **1**(1), 30–36.

Gardner, G., Carryer, J., Dunn, S.V., Gardner, A. (2004). *Nurse Practitioner Standards Project.* Queensland University of Technology: Australian Nursing Council.

Hanson, C.M. (2005). Understanding regulatory, legal, and credentialing requirements. In A.B. Hamric, J.A. Spross, C.M. Hanson (Eds) *Advanced practice nursing. An integrative approach* (3rd Edition), pp. 781–808. St Louis: Elsevier Saunders.

Henderson, J.P. (1999). The National Commission for Certifying Agencies. In A. Cary, C. Wharton (Eds) *Quality assurance through credentialing: Volume 2 – Concepts, issues and trends,* pp. 37–41. Washington: American Nurses Credentialing Centre.

International Council of Nurses. (1986). *Report on the regulation of nursing: A report on the present. A position for the future.* Geneva: Author.

International Council of Nurses. (1997). *An approval system for schools of nursing. Guidelines.* Geneva: Author.

International Council of Nurses. (2005). *Guidelines on shaping effective health policies.* Geneva: Author. Retrieved 1 October, 2005 from http://www.icn.ch/guidelines.htm

International Council of Nurses Credentialing Forum. (2004). *Japan country report.* Unpublished.

International Council of Nurses Credentialing Forum. (2005). *Ireland country report.* Unpublished.

International Council of Nurses & World Health Organization. (2005). *Nursing regulation: A futures perspective.* Geneva. Retrieved 14/7/05 from http://icn.ch/regactivities. htm#position

International HIV/AIDS Alliance. (2002.) *Advocacy in Action: A toolkit to support NGOs and CBOs responding to HIV/AIDS.* Brighton: Author.

Kim, D.D. (2003). *The APN in Korea.* Presented at the ICN Conference, Geneva, 2003.

Lewis, C., Smolenski, M.C. (2000). Practice credentials, licensure, approval of practice, certification, and privileging. In J.V. Hickey, R.M. Ouimette, S.L. Venegoni (Eds) *Advanced practice nursing. Changing roles and clinical applications* (2nd Edition), pp. 66–81. Philadelphia: Lippincott.

National Association of Clinical Nursing Specialists. (2003). NACNS position paper: Regulatory credentialing of clinical nurse specialists. *Clinical Nurse Specialist,* **17**(3), 163–169.

National Council for the Professional Development of Nursing and Midwifery. (2001). *Framework for the establishment of advanced nurse practitioner and advanced midwifery practitioner posts.* Dublin: Author.

National Council for the Professional Development of Nursing and Midwifery. (2004). *Framework for the establishment of advanced nurse practitioner and advanced midwife practitioner posts* (2nd Edition). Dublin: Author. Retrieved March 6, 2006 from http://www.ncnm.ie/files/ANP%20Framework.pdf

National Council of State Boards of Nursing. (1993). *Regulation of advanced nursing practice: NCSBN position.* Retrieved 8 July, 2005 from www.ncsbn.org

National Council of State Boards of Nursing. (2002). *Regulation of advanced practice nursing: 2002 National Council of State Boards of Nursing position paper.* Retrieved 8 July, 2005 from www.ncsbn.org

New Zealand Nurses Organization. (Undated). *NZNO certification: Nurse clinician.* Retrieved July 5, 2005 from http://www.nzno.org.nz/Site/Professional/ANP/default.aspx

Nurses Board of Victoria (NBV). (2004). *Process for nurse practitioner endorsement.* Melbourne: Author.

Nursing and Midwifery Council (NMC). (2005). *Consultation on a framework for the standard for post-registration nursing.* London, Author.

Nursing Council of New Zealand (NCNZ). (2002). *Nurse practitioner endorsement: Guidelines for applicants.* Wellington: Author.

Nurses Registration Board of New South Wales (NRB). (2002). *Guidelines for educational institutions wishing to submit for approval in regard to authorisation of nurse practitioners.* Retrieved 20 July, 2005 from http://www.nursesreg.nsw.gov.au/np_cours.pdf

Nurses Registration Board of New South Wales (NRB). (2003). *Nurse practitioners in New South Wales.* Retrieved June 15, 2005 from www.nmb.nsw.gov.au/np_info.pdf

Porcher, F.K. (2003). Licensure, certification and credentialing. In M.D. Mezey, D.O. McGivern, E.M. Sullivan-Marx (Eds) *Nurse practitioners. Evolution of advanced practice* (4th Edition), pp. 415–430. New York: Springer.

Professional Regulation Commission, Board of Nursing, Manila. (2002). *Nursing specialty certification program. BON Res. No.14S.1999 and guidelines for implementation.* Manila: Author.

Pulcini, J., Wagner, M. (2004). *Nurse practitioner education in the United States.* Retrieved April 24, 2005 from http://icn-apnetwork.org/

Royal College of Nursing. (2002, revised 2005). *Nurse practitioner: An RCN guide to the nurse practitioner role, competencies and programme approval.* London: Author.

Sharma, R.R. (Undated). *An introduction to advocacy. Training guide.* Washington: SARA Project–Advocacy Academy for Educational Development.

Singapore Ministry of Health. (2005). *The Nurses & Midwives (Amendment) Bill.* Retrieved 8 July, 2005 from http://www.moh.gov.sg/corp/about/newsroom/speeches/details.do?id=31227981

Styles, M.M. (1999). Credentialing as a global profession in progress: Part 1: Measuring up. In A. Cary, C. Wharton (Eds) *Quality assurance through credentialing: Volume 1 – Global perspectives.* Washington: American Nurses Credentialing Centre.

Styles, M.M., Affara, F.A. (1997). *ICN on regulation: Towards a 21st century model.* Geneva: International Council of Nurses.

Tarrant, F. & Associates. (2005). *Literature review of nurse practitioner legislation and regulation.* Canadian Nurse Practitioner Initiative. Retrieved 24 June, 2005 from http://www.cnpi.ca/documents/pdf/Legislation_Regulation_Literature_Review_e.pdf

Trans Atlantic Consumer Dialogue (TACD). (2000). *Briefing paper on mutual recognition agreements (MRAs).* Retrieved on 3 October, 2005 from http://www.tacd.org/cgi-bin/db.cgi?page=view&config=admin/docs.cfg&id=193

Chapter 5
Education for advanced nursing practice

Introduction

The credibility and sustainability of practice is rooted in the type of educational preparation the advanced practice nurse (APN) undergoes. As advanced nursing roles emerge, defining educational preparation at an advanced enough level provides a basis from which to differentiate this level of practice from that of the generalist nurse. National nursing associations, credentialing bodies, regulatory authorities, governmental agencies and ministries of health all play a part in establishing standards for education that contribute to legitimatising the advanced nursing roles.

At the start of new initiatives, flexible developmental educational options rather than those of a prescriptive nature appear to be more beneficial as they allow for continual review, evaluation and contextual adaptation of educational requirements. At this stage you may find nurses who are able to work as an APN without graduate level qualifications, but who have acquired competencies for this type of practice through appropriate experience and completion of specified accredited or approved courses.

Educational issues affecting advanced nursing practice are multifactorial and multidimensional. Educators face challenges all the way from creating to sustaining advanced nursing programmes that prepare the graduate for various settings in current and future health systems. Students and graduates in any learning endeavour will practise increasingly in an interdisciplinary or multidisciplinary manner; thus education has to take up the task of educating for working in partnership and through collaborative practice models (Schober & McKay, 2004). Difficulties facing educators working to graduate skilled and knowledgeable APNs include: decreasing financial resources; faculty shortages or faculties ill equipped to educate APNs; lack of available and poorly suited clinical sites; limited exposure to good role models or mentors; and an over-crowded curriculum.

Characteristics of advanced nursing practice education

ICN (2005) recognises that scope of practice and standards as well as opportunities for education will vary from nation to nation. The health care needs of the world's populations, as well as resources allocated, influence progress and the direction of educational development. Historically and up to the present time, educational qualifications for the APN role varied from the awarding of certificates for post-basic courses to undertaking a formal university programme and obtaining a masters degree. An ICN official position on the definition of advanced nursing practice recommends educational preparation at masters level.

Regardless of the sequence of role development in a country or locale, an educational mandate that reflects a well-defined scope of practice is pivotal for establishing relevant educational programmes. The curriculum, courses and course content will be driven by the scope of practice and the context in which advanced practice is developing. The authors refer the reader to Chapter 2 for a discussion of issues influencing definition of scope of practice.

Central to establishing the direction for advanced nursing practice education are the educational institutions and programmes recognised by accrediting or approving bodies. Consistent with ICN's vision of 21st century regulatory models (Styles & Affara, 1997) and the work by the International Nurse Practitioner/Advanced Practice Nursing Network (INP/APNN) standards for education include the following:

(1) Programmes prepare the generalist nurse for practice beyond that expected for entry into generalist nursing practice, and include opportunities for the student to gain knowledge, experience and the necessary skills to competently function in an advanced role.

(2) Programmes prepare the nurse to practise in the health care environment of a country to the fullest extent of the role as defined in the recognised scope of practice.

(3) Qualified faculty staff the programmes.

(4) Programmes are accredited by the authorised credentialing body.

(5) Programmes facilitate lifelong learning and maintenance of competencies.
     (ICN, 2005)

The case for masters level education

There appears to be strong international support for masters level preparation
for advanced nursing practice. Castledine (2003) stresses that a *clinically based
masters degree* is the foundation for advanced practice education (p. 11).
Inman (2003) agrees with this view, and notes that this recommendation is understandable considering that an APN is expected to demonstrate expert clinical
performance that is accompanied by a high level of professional attributes such
as critical decision-making and leadership skills.

The International Council of Nurses (2002; 2005), national nursing organisations and national task forces that have studied this issue (An Bord Altranis,
2003; Canadian Nurses Association [CNA], 2002; Gardner *et al.*, 2004; Maclaine
et al., 2004; National Taskforce on Quality Nurse Practitioner Education
[NTF], 2002; Nursing Council New Zealand [NCNZ], 2002) recommend or
require masters level preparation or its equivalent. Key informants (personal
communication) from Australia, Canada, France, Hong Kong, Netherlands, New
Zealand, Philippines, Singapore, Switzerland, Taiwan and the United States
consider a masters degree best demonstrates the academic progression needed
to move from generalist nurse education to the advanced level of knowledge
required by the APN.

One aspect of gaining credibility for advanced nursing practice is through
obtaining convincing educational credentials. Nurses themselves will need to
recognise that, ideally, advanced practice requires a masters qualification. At a
practical level, other health care professionals, administrators and policy
makers must be informed and persuaded as to the fundamental standard for
APN education. When APNs attain consensus that education must take place
at graduate level, it will be possible to convince professionals, administrators and
policy makers that this is the standard of education for advanced practice.

Debate around masters level education

In describing the forty-year history of nurse practitioner (NP) development in
the United States, Towers (2005) writes that education evolved from at first
being a post-registered nurse certificate to eventually reaching masters degree level.
Initial NP courses were commonly offered as continuing education components
at universities, hospitals, medical schools and schools of nursing. Over time
curricula became more refined with inclusion of increased course and clinical
requirements. Now a masters degree is considered the entry-level requirement
for advanced nursing practice in the United States. Currently there is active

discussion around the need to establish a clinical doctorate to provide a higher level of preparation for those nurses who want to remain in clinical practice (American Association of Colleges of Nursing [AACN], 2004; key informants, personal communication). Educational progress has evolved in response to service needs as well as educational developments throughout the entire country. Over the years standardisation of educational programmes in the United States has been accomplished through the work and consensus of national nursing associations resulting in the identification of quality indicators and requirements for programme accreditation (NTF, 2002; key informants, personal communication).

Setting masters level education as the entry level into advanced nursing practice, however, may simply be unrealistic in the beginning phase of integration of this role into the health care workforce. Inadequate human and financial resources, limited opportunities for nursing education, the absence of properly prepared faculty, and the newness and poor recognition of nursing as a profession in a nation diminish the possibility of reaching this standard. In addition, other factors such as competing health care priorities suggest that strategies for introducing and evolving advanced practice education require innovative thinking, flexibility, and the willingness and ability to plan over a long period. What may be important in the initial stages of introduction and implementation of new advanced nursing roles is to set masters level education as a standard to attain rather than as an immediate requirement.

Country variations in educational philosophy, approach and development

The initial Family Nurse Practitioner programme established in Botswana in 1981 focused on the comprehensive primary health care (PHC) needs of the country with emphasis on assessment, diagnosis and management of common diseases, health promotion and disease prevention. The programme designed for registered nurses and midwives has progressed from one year to 18 months in length and includes clinical components usually found in masters programmes as described by other countries. External examiners have consistently given the programme high marks, as well as a recommendation to offer it at the masters level (Seitio, 2000; key informant, personal communication).

Similarly, in Samoa advanced nursing programmes were developed with support by the World Health Organization (WHO) to meet the country's needs in PHC. Following a period when nurses were educated in New Zealand, the decision was made to initiate an advanced practice programme in Samoa utilising external nursing and physician consultants and local doctors. The education provided resulted in a focus on using a medical approach to clinical practice. The programme was one year long and then evolved to 18 months with the addition of core courses and more options. Since 1993, forty nurses have undertaken the Advanced Diploma Programme and earned the title of nurse consultants. These nurses, now able to do health assessment, clinical decision-making and diagnosing, work in health care settings throughout the country, mostly in community settings without doctors. Critical to future advanced nursing practice development in this country is the move of nursing education to the university with an undergraduate degree now the basic entry level for nursing in Samoa (I. Enoka, personal communication).

In a continued effort to promote a national approach for advanced nursing practice, the Canadian Nurses Association (2002) having acknowledged the uneven development of educational programmes in the country, hope to promote a coordinated effort by providing a national framework for advanced nursing practice. An integral part of this framework is a synchronised effort to move toward graduate level education, while at the same time recognising the uniqueness of the Canadian health care system. A comparative competency analysis from 2002 to 2004 was conducted as part of the Canadian Nurse Practitioner Initiative [CPNI] (2004). Consensus was achieved on national core competencies for the NP with the expectation that this would provide a basis for sound programme development as well as a pan-Canadian licensure/registration examination for nurse practitioners. While this initiative appears to be focused on the NP in PHC, it should be noted that Canada also has had a presence of mainly hospital based CNS since the 1980s, the majority of whom have had graduate level education (key informants, personal communication). It is hoped that a national framework will promote consistency and clarity for advanced nursing practice in Canada.

In the United Kingdom the Royal College of Nursing (RCN) developed the first NP course in 1990 and currently approves NP programmes at both bachelors and masters level for nine higher education institutions through the RCN Accreditation Unit. A National Organisation of Nurse Practitioner Faculties – United Kingdom, based on the United States model, was established in 2001, not only to promote quality education, but also to connect representatives from the RCN approved and non-RCN approved programmes that provide undergraduate and postgraduate education for nurses. Through internal and external consultation the professional organisation has established 15 educational standards and criteria that higher education institutions must meet to receive approved status. In an attempt to promote common teaching content for the UK, the educational standards and criteria are connected to an agreed-upon core of knowledge and skills (Maclaine, 2004; RCN, 2002).

The four countries comprising the United Kingdom have progressed toward masters level NP education at a different momentum. Although a bachelors NP programme was eventually closed in Scotland, nurses can now access two advanced practice masters programmes, one of which has been approved by the RCN. Wales has bachelors level NP programmes, but these are being phased out in order to move toward masters level education. Northern Ireland had an RCN approved NP programme offered by its Institute in Northern Ireland, but the programme lost this approval when it transferred to a university setting. Nurse practitioner education is not thriving in Northern Ireland owing to an excess of doctors. It appears that the key to the success of Scotland and Wales in offering university level advanced practice education lies in the fact that entry level education for the generalist nurse is a bachelors degree, unlike in England where basic nursing education has stayed at the diploma level. The prospect of an all-graduate nursing workforce, combined with efforts to modernise the health system by establishing a national career framework which recognises advanced practice as requiring a masters level education, may partially account for Scotland and Wales offering the masters degree sooner than England (Skills for Health, 2005; K. Maclaine, personal communication). As in the United States, there is a move in the United Kingdom and Ireland to promote clinical doctorate preparation in nursing. Institutions have recognised and identified an opportunity to prepare nurses as clinical leaders in a complex and changing health care culture (McKenna & Cutcliffe, 2001; University of Stirling, undated).

The Nursing Council of New Zealand's [NCNZ] (2002) framework for NP endorsement stipulated at the outset that a clinically focused masters education, or its equivalent, is required for entry into practice. The Nursing Council approved masters degree includes theory, research and clinical practice hours. It is mandatory that the NP takes additional approved pharmacology courses relative to their specialty if the prescribing option is to be exercised.

In Australia the advanced nursing practice presence and thus education has developed independently by state or territory. Mutual acceptance of a number of educational programmes across state or territory boundaries exists. Not all universities in Australia are developing courses specifically for APNs, but many are offering a range of programmes that can be combined to achieve masters level education (key informants, personal communication). In New South Wales (NSW) a nurse applying for authorisation as an NP must provide evidence of successful completion of a masters degree approved by the NSW Nurses Registration Board (NRB), or provide a package of evidence fulfilling Board requirements (NMB of NSW, 2005). Similarly, in Victoria the Nursing Board is responsible for accrediting masters level courses and the therapeutic medication management modules that are necessary for NP endorsement (State Government of Victoria, 2005).

The Nurse Practitioner Standards project sponsored by the Australian Nursing and Midwifery Council and NCNZ (Gardner *et al.*, 2004) has provided data and advice for New Zealand and Australia that include standards of education for advanced nursing practice, to enable them to develop a dual country recognition system required to meet the provisions of the Trans Tasman Mutual Recognition Act 1977. There is mutual agreement by both countries that a masters degree is the minimum education level for NPs.

The World Health Organization-South East Asia Region ([WHO-SEAR] (2003), in making the case for a flexible global nursing and midwifery workforce, suggests that professionals, when well-educated, can be more fully utilised in diverse settings. WHO-SEAR provides a conceptual framework to assist countries to develop strategies that assure a strong and effective nursing and midwifery workforce with the proper knowledge, skills and attitudes to fit the health care setting. The emphasis of this approach is on strong coordination between education and practice with service needs driving educational decision-making.

- Joint appointments in education and practice settings.
- Joint (education and service) planning committee to assess overall service needs.
- Advisory committees for education programmes that consist of both nursing/midwifery educators as well as clinical nurses/midwives.
- Joint research between educators and clinicians.
- Shared continuing education for nurses/midwives, educators and clinicians.
- Possible renewable license based on evidence of continuing and maintenance and enhancement of clinical competency

Figure 5.1   Recommendations for coordination of nursing education development. (Source: WHO-SEAR, 2003.)

This is seen as the best way to achieve goals of increasing equity and accessibility of services. The view is presented that if an educational programme is not led by service needs, tension can develop when skills and competencies do not correspond with service requirements and health priorities.

WHO-SEAR makes a number of recommendations for countries to consider in strengthening the coordination of educational development for nursing. Refer to Figure 5.1 for these recommendations.

Paths of entry into programmes and length of study

As advanced nursing practice develops internationally, requirements for specific educational preparation, as well as the length of these programmes, vary. Study may consist of updating courses with the intention of refining generalist nursing skills, to programmes with restrictive entry requirements for programme completion. Table 5.1 provides examples of the range of options available globally in terms of entry requirements, length of study, qualification obtained, or title. The diversity of approach to advanced nursing practice education is further portrayed in country vignettes. These examples also show how sensitive the nature of development is to the nature of the opportunities available in the context in which the role is evolving.

Vignettes of advanced nursing practice educational development

Vignettes 5.1 to 5.3 illustrate different approaches taken to prepare nurses for the advanced practice role. Timor Leste, a country faced with serious and urgent health care needs and a shortage of adequately prepared nurses and doctors, needed to train nurses with advanced practice skills quickly. Wuhan University in China illustrates a step-by-step plan of integrating advanced nursing practice into the higher education sector, while the French example shows how nurses have used a projected shortage of health care providers to promote the concept of APNs educated to a masters level.

Table 5.1 Advanced nursing practice programmes listed by entry requirements, length of study and title earned. (Sources: Key Informants, personal communication; WHO-Western Pacific Region, [WHO-WPR], 2001, 16–17.)

Country	Entry Criteria	Length of Programme	Result
Australia	Graduate certificate + experience + courses BSN	24–72 months depending on full time or part time status (2 months for medication module)	Diploma or title MSN
Bahrain	A.D. BSc.	9–18 months depending on entry criteria	Diploma (post-basic in specialised area)
Botswana	RN with good passes at Cambridge level	18 months	Diploma
Canada	Variable	Variable (post-diploma, undergraduate or graduate levels)	Diploma BSN MSN
Hong Kong	BSN	3 years part-time	MSN
Iceland	Not available	24 months	MSN
Ireland	Not available	24 months	MSN
Japan	Not available	24 months	MSN, Certification
Macau	BD or above	24 months	Specialised Nurse
Netherlands	BSN + experience	2 years	MSN
New Zealand	Undergraduate degree in nursing or equivalent	24 months	MSN or MSN equivalent portfolio
Pakistan	BScN, Min. GPA, Interview, English Proficiency Exam	2 years full-time	MScN
Republic of South Africa	RN	12 months post-basic	Specialist
Singapore	BSN Advanced diploma nursing specialty	18 months	MSN
Sweden	RN + experience + right to prescribe	18–24 months	MSN after full 24 months; ANP after 18 months
Switzerland	Matura (Gymnasium final degree) Clinical Experience TOEFL English exam	36 months (minimum)	MSN

Table 5.1   *(cont'd)*

Country	Entry Criteria	Length of Programme	Result
Taiwan	BSN	4 months 2 years	Certification MSN
Thailand	Not available	24 months	Certification Masters
United Kingdom	Clinical experience	2–3 years usually part time	BSN MSN
United States	BSN, Minimum GPA, GRE or Miller Analogy Test, reference letters, scholarly writing, interview, clinical experience as RN	18–24 months	MSN or post-masters certificate
Western Pacific	Post-registration as general nurse	At least one year (varies among the islands)	Nurse Practitioner Nurse Specialist (titles vary)

Vignette 5.1   Advanced nursing practice education responding to urgent health care needs in Timor-Leste.

Lack of doctors and properly educated nurses led to the development of the Advanced Practice Training Programme (APNT) in Timor-Leste in 2002. The object-ive of the programme was to assist nurses gain the knowledge and skills to make independent diagnoses, manage the associated diseases, and provide disease prevention interventions in rural areas without doctors. The Minister of Health in conjunction with WHO developed a need-based programme to educate nurses to perform health histories, physical examinations, diagnoses, treatment, coun-selling and health promotion for diseases and conditions common to Timor-Leste. The six-month competency-based programme includes theory and clinical prac-tice with distance learning options. During this time of transition when the need is urgent 'Clinical Nurses' provide competent services with confidence. The APNT is a cost-effective and practical strategy to address an urgent need for preventative and curative health care services.

(WHO, 2005)

Assessment of prior experience and bridging mechanisms

Introduction of advanced practice-like services at times precedes identifica-tion of scope of practice, core competencies and educational programmes, as well as regulation of the professional role. A lag often occurs between the reality of practice already in place and subsequent support from the regulatory and education institutions. This sequence in establishing advanced nursing practice

---

Vignette 5.2   Emerging APN university-based master's education in China.

Wuhan University signed an agreement with Project Hope in 2001 requesting assistance to establish a School of Nursing in an academic setting rather than a hospital. Active support by the president of the university, along with an interest in meeting international standards for nursing education further facilitated this initiative. The 2003 approved curriculum for a masters level programme required that 1/3 of required courses are similar to those taken by other university students, 1/3 are elective courses and 1/3 are in a declared major. The aim is to educate graduates who are clinically competent and critical decision-makers. Following consultation with clinical staff in hospitals, the newly created curriculum simultaneously integrates theory and clinical practice. As judged by experience with the first group of students, it has been a success.

An objective of the programme is to have a clinical focus with a research thesis that deals with clinical practice issues. In 2006 Wuhan University plans to begin to develop a clinically-focused doctoral programme intended to prepare nurses for advanced nursing practice-like roles. Exposure of leaders in Beijing to models in the United States has inspired interest in promoting advanced nursing roles in community health and other specialties throughout China. Wuhan University functions directly under the Ministry of Education and has the potential of developing a new model for nursing education and practice with advanced nursing practice characteristics that can be adopted nationwide. Of note in the developmental process of this initiative is the presence of a Dean for the School of Nursing with over 15 years of working in China, as well as experience with advanced nursing practice roles, undergraduate and graduate programmes in the United States.

(M. Petrini, personal communication)

---

can contribute to creating a less than favourable environment for sound role development as it often leads to uneven processes for education, the establishment of variable entry requirements, and difficulties in identifying and implementing realistic clinical practicum experiences for students.

In locations where nurses acquire extensive clinical experience prior to receiving any formal education, a mechanism is needed that acknowledges prior knowledge and skills and satisfies education and regulatory authorities. For instance, a nurse may be asked to present a well-organised profile of experience, or a portfolio, as well as undertake specified courses to bridge the gap in order to attain the equivalence of a masters qualification. In this way it is possible to fully utilise the already existing potential in the nursing workforce (Castledine, 2005; Gardner *et al.*, 2004; NCNZ, 2002; key informants, personal communication).

Curriculum development

In planning a curriculum supportive of advanced nursing practice, defining fundamental elements of the anticipated content and level of education is essential. In addition to taking into account the current status of the generalist role, advanced

---

Vignette 5.3   Promoting advanced nursing education in France.

Nursing in France is considered to be a sub-discipline of medicine. The French Act (promulgated initially in 1980 and revised in 1984, 1993, 2002 and 2004) must be approved by the Academy of Medicine before its adoption by the Parliament. Even though nurse anaesthetists are recognised, nurses in this role legally work under the supervision of an anaesthesiologist. Nursing education has remained non-academic with a history of physicians teaching nursing students. In 2003 the Ministry of Health requested a report on the consequences of the medical short-age on health care services in France. Two reports indicated that some medical services needed to be delegated to nonmedical professionals. The French Nurses Association (ANFIDE) anticipated this by informing nurses about advanced practice. A press campaign was launched to provide information related to the introduction of advanced nursing practice in France, its regulation, account-ability, educational requirement and salary. Inspired by the introduction of advanced practice in the province of Quebec (Canada), ANFIDE recommended that educational preparation of the clinical nurse specialists with advanced practice privileges should be at masters degree level. A first set of pilot studies was launched in 2004 to assess the feasibility of the recommendations. A second set of pilot studies will be conducted in 2005. ANFIDE remains proactive in promoting the introduction of advanced practice in France with a level of education that creates 'maxi nurses' not 'mini doctors'.

(C. Debout, personal communication)

---

practice programmes must be strongly rooted in the scope of practice identified for APN roles. It is also important to have faculty, staff and instructors who understand the scope of practice and subsequent requirements for advanced nursing education, and have the expertise to undertake curriculum and programme development. Institutions lacking faculty capable of carrying out this task may have to utilise expertise from nations with experience to fill the gaps while national faculty develop the necessary competence in this area. Collaborative partnerships with experienced institutions, use of knowledgeable consultants and accessing the growing number of resources in this area are strategies to promote self-reliance and sustainability of new programmes (key informants, personal communication). Figure 5.2 identifies important points to consider or necessary actions to take in programme and curriculum development.

A curriculum framework to promote flexibility

Figure 5.3 suggests a framework for curriculum development. The framework includes three conceptual cornerstones developed by Gagan *et al.* (2002) in a model for curriculum revision. They are health policy, community needs and demands, and curriculum goals.

Constant interface among the three cornerstones creates a dynamic environment that updates curriculum development by promoting ongoing reflection on the pertinence of the educational programme to the external environment.

- Identify and define need or opportunity for advanced nursing practice.
- Appraise the anticipated APN scope of practice.
- Assess the role parameters and identify the locales where the advanced practice nurse will practise in the health system. Will graduates be able to practise to the extent of their educational preparation?
- Explore any regulatory or policy issues that may affect recognition of graduates.
- Assess the need and secure short term and long term human and financial resources in order to decide if it is feasible to start and sustain the programme.
- Make available a level of advanced education that is realistic considering the country's needs and the availability of human and financial resources.
- Develop a definitive curriculum and programme management document.
- Establish criteria and a plan for recruiting faculty for the short term.
- Develop strategies to recruit and educate faculty for the long term.
- Set up criteria for entry into the programme.
- Limit the number of students to suit to a realistic faculty/student ratio and available clinical sites. Starting with a smaller number of students allows for a closer evaluation of the programme.
- Identify the possibilities for advanced clinical practicum sites and negotiate how they will be used.
- Create a framework for periodic review and evaluation of the programme to allow for adjustment and progressive development as the role matures and the health and education contexts change.

Figure 5.2 Points to consider in programme and curriculum development. (Source: ICN 2005; Key Informants, personal communication; NTF, 2002.)

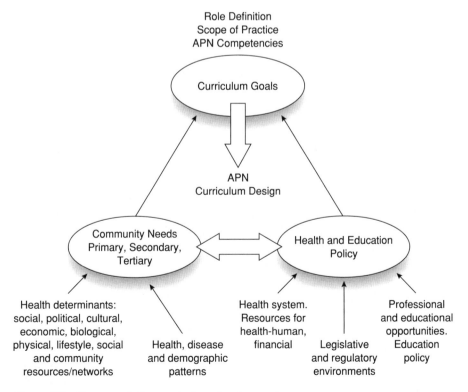

Figure 5.3 Framework for curriculum development.

Frequent contributions from students, graduates and faculty allow for a continuing assessment of graduates' abilities to meet health care service needs for populations and communities within the realities and opportunities of the health care environment. It should be noted that role definition, scope of practice and APN competencies are considered to be the foundation for identifying curriculum goals.

The context for care will shape the range, focus, content and quality of practice and services, and consequently the scope of practice and competencies needed by the APN. Figure 5.3 demonstrates the multiple factors in the environment that can impinge and influence curriculum goals and educational outcomes. These factors include:

- The determinants of health derived from a model of health developed by Dahlgren and Whitehead (1991) that suggests that health status is a result of a complex interface among an individual's age, sex and hereditary factors, individual lifestyles, social and community networks
- Health, illness and demographic patterns
- The regulatory environment
- Resources for health – human and financial
- Professional education and opportunities for post-basic and continuing education
- Health systems, especially policies and the health system structure affecting health care priorities and goals, funding for and access to health services.

Conceptually the framework is congruent with the established curriculum guidelines of the National Organization of Nurse Practitioner Faculties (NONPF, 2000) and the American Association of Colleges of Nursing (AACN, 1996).

Curriculum: course distribution

Core courses in the curriculum form the foundation for advanced nursing practice programmes. Course content should be derived from the level of advanced practice implicit within the scope that defines the services to be provided by programme graduates. Identifying essential core courses at a national level will help to promote consistency in APN education offered within a country. Hopefully in the future, it will be possible to reach international consensus on core courses thus beginning to promote consistency not only within nations but across borders.

Figure 5.4 illustrates how core courses may fall into two categories. The first deals with the essential theoretical basis of advanced nursing practice, while the second focuses on the essential clinical components. A third group of courses prepares the APN for in-depth practice in a field. These courses may vary as they will be tailored to specific areas e.g. epidemiology, infectious disease control, health education, informatics, or specific roles e.g. maternal–child health, mental health, oncology, community health (AACN, 1996; key informants,

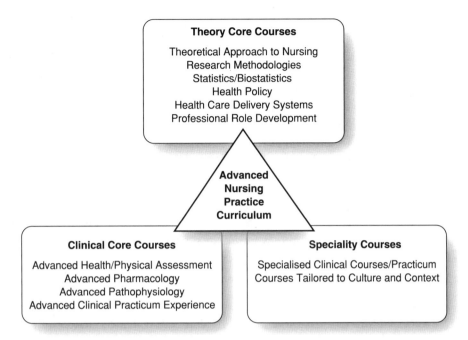

Figure 5.4 Advanced practice curriculum: course distribution. (Source: AACN, 1996; Key Informants, personal communication.)

personal communication). Key informants emphasise the importance of making available courses that address health care needs specific to the country.

It is expected that each country or region will modify the curriculum in order to be consistent with the mission of the programme as well as the health care needs and priorities. In surveying 14 programmes in Australia and New Zealand the type of courses varied but study of pharmacology, research and advanced assessment were common to all (Gardner *et al.*, 2004). Courses described in masters programmes in Pakistan, Hong Kong, Taiwan, Singapore, Sweden, Australia and New Zealand are consistent with the curriculum design described in Figure 5.4 (AACN 1996; Aga Khan University School of Nursing, 2004; Hong Kong Polytechnic University, 2004; National University of Singapore, 2005; NTF, 2002; University of Skövde, 2003; key informants, personal communication;). It must be stressed that a variety of resources should be reviewed and considered when initiating and developing appropriate advanced nursing practice curriculum. See Appendix 5 for examples of course descriptions and the resource section for assistance in educational programme development.

Advanced practice clinical experience

'Clinical experience can be defined as providing "direct" client care to individuals, families, and or communities' (NONPF, 1995, p. 77). Clinical learning and practical clinical experiences are significant components of advanced practice education (Gardner *et al.*, 2004; key informants, personal communication). Identifying and providing relevant clinical experience challenges both established programmes and new initiatives. Key informants familiar with pioneer programmes admit initially there is reliance on physicians to teach clinical course components, while qualified nursing faculty teach nursing courses. Over time a blending of these efforts leads to interdisciplinary teaching approaches for the theoretical elements of the programme and in the clinical practicum. In planning classroom-based courses that prepare for clinical experience, consideration should be given to the availability of adequate physical space, demonstration models, clinical simulation experience, and access to audiovisual aids, computer and information technology and library resources. It is admitted that where resources are limited, the ingenuity and the creativity of the educator will be stretched in providing quality education (key informants, personal communication).

Settings for clinical experience

Clinical settings should be sufficiently diverse to ensure that the student will meet educational objectives. Sites need to be evaluated periodically for the quality of learning offered and to ensure that they are not overburdened by excessive numbers of students (NTF, 2002). Success in meeting clinical learning objectives entails exposure to a variety of clinicians and experiences. The main way of facilitating clinical learning in advanced nursing practice education is through the use of preceptors. The Canadian Nurses Association (2004) defines preceptorship as:

> *a formal, one-to-one relationship of pre-determined length, between an experienced nurse (preceptor) and a novice (preceptee) designed to assist the novice in successfully adjusting to a new role. The novice may be a student or an already practising nurse moving into a new role, domain or setting.*

Preceptors are not always nurses, and in settings where physicians are preceptors and unaccustomed to being evaluated by nurses, on-site visits and assessment will need to be approached diplomatically to ensure that the quality of clinical experience they will provide meets programme expectations, while at the same time showing appreciation for their support and interest.

Clinical practice facilitated by preceptors provides students with opportunities to conduct history taking, perform physical assessments, diagnose and manage acute as well as chronic illnesses, provide health promotion interventions, develop case management skills, and make referrals to appropriate resources in a supervised learning environment. Students entering a specialty area of study for clinical learning are scheduled according to their background, interest in the specialty, and availability of qualified preceptors in the specialty. Criteria for clinical experience hours can be established either within the definitive documents of a programme, or by the credentialing system practised by a state, province or country. It has been the experience of the authors that there is a tendency for new programmes to plan clinical practicums that are for the most part observational. Limiting clinical experience to this form of learning does not allow students to develop the level of clinical competence that is the hallmark of a role grounded in direct clinical care.

Doucette *et al.* (2005) in describing difficulties in arranging clinical practice sites for primary health care nurse practitioner students, lists challenges in establishing sites for clinical experience. They include:

- Competition for clinical sites with medical students
- Different role requirements for rural, remote and urban settings
- Limited appropriate clinical sites
- Lack of understanding of advanced nursing practice competencies
- Poor communication of expected clinical learning outcomes
- Uncertain and uneven quality of precepting and mentoring.

Key informants (personal communication) and observations during clinical site visits by the authors were consistent with the experiences described by Doucette *et al.* (2005). One way to alleviate some of these problems is to develop agreements or contracts clarifying expectations and responsibilities with agencies or individuals providing the clinical learning experiences. Frequently in the initial stages, verbal rather than written agreement allows for flexibility as each party concerned learns the possibilities, limitations and expectations of the clinical setting. Agreements should address topics such as anticipated results of the clinical attachment, faculty and preceptor responsibilities, liability insurance, as well as specific areas of local concern, or actions required to assure patient safety. For example, in Hong Kong, following the experience of the city of SARS, students are required to provide evidence of completion of an infectious disease workshop prior to any clinical assignment. Having preceptors well orientated to the clinical learning needs of the APN student adds considerably to making the clinical practicum experience a success.

Preceptors and quality of clinical placements

Fundamental to advanced nursing practice education is the recognition that the nature of the clinical assessment and care management APNs carry out differs from that done by the generalist nurse. Advanced practitioners are prepared to carry out more detailed data collection, often including extensive physical examination. In addition, the APN will be required to apply advanced skills in synthesising information from this expanded clinical assessment. An ability to use effective clinical reasoning and decision-making is essential since the capacity to evaluate information impacts on decisions made for safe and effective care (Taylor-Seehafer *et al.*, 2004). A critical feature of a clinical practicum is the quality of the opportunities provided for students to learn assessment and care management skills, and demonstrate these in a real life clinical setting.

The quality of clinical learning is intimately linked to the skill, experience, expertise and characteristics of faculty and the designated clinical preceptor (Inman, 2003; NTF, 2002; Spross, 2005). Preceptors and faculty must have an appropriate background and education to function in this role. O'Malley *et al.* (2000)

identify experience and expertise in the clinical field combined with leadership, communication, decision-making skills, a desire to teach and an ability to be adaptable to the learners as qualities to look for in a preceptor. Various methods can be used to assess the qualifications of a potential preceptor. ICN (2005) advises preparation of faculty at a level equal to, or above, that of the students. Verification of credentials and *curriculum vitae* is needed when identifying faculty or preceptors and when assigning students for clinical attachment. A site visit and interview with preceptors is desirable and will help to assess the appropriateness of the site. It provides an opportunity to ensure there is common understanding of the practicum requirements. Providing a list of clinical competencies and expectations for student performance gives guidance on the level of competence expected of programme graduates (NTF, 2002). Clearly defined student and preceptor responsibilities (Table 5.2) are useful in making clinical learning relevant.

As mentioned earlier, when programmes are first introduced physicians are often asked to teach clinical reasoning and skills. One way to ensure that the preceptor is aware of the APN focus is to provide written preceptor guidelines that are consistent with the programme goals for the advanced clinical practicum. Examples of preceptor guidelines are provided in Appendix 6, and the resource section indicates where more information can be obtained on mentoring and preceptorship. Over time as more qualified nursing faculty and preceptors become available, reliance on physicians can be decreased.

Planning for the precepting experience

Ideally the potential preceptor should assess his or her interest and ability to find the time to teach as well as serve as a clinical instructor for the student. Taking time to assess the required responsibilities and setting before committing to the preceptor role is important for success. Factors such as patient load, space limitations and other time commitments need to be taken account of and be explicitly built into the practicum experience if it is to be of mutual benefit and cause minimal disruptions to the work and routines of the site. At the beginning of the clinical attachment, the student and preceptor need to confirm what clinical objectives are to be attained, and clarify each other's expectations of the experience. Also, mutually acceptable times and dates for the practicum need to discussed and agreed to. Upon completion of the practicum and using a formal evaluation process, preceptor and student are encouraged to review the clinical learning outcomes and document strengths, weaknesses and recommendations. Refer to Appendix 5 for examples of student and preceptor evaluation forms.

Examples of APN student practicum in new settings

Vignettes 5.4 and 5.5 describe instances where APN student practicum was initiated in settings that had no prior experience with the APN role or APN

Table 5.2 Preceptor and student responsibilities in advanced clinical practicum. (Source: University of South Carolina, 2005; AACN, 1996.)

Preceptor's Responsibility	Student's Responsibility
Student objectives as well as the background and expertise of the preceptor will guide preceptor responsibilities. Common responsibilities expected of a preceptor can include the following: (1) Select patients and provide learning experiences appropriate to clinical objectives of the student (2) Observe the student directly and provide constructive advice (3) Schedule consultation with the student to review patient history, physical exam, diagnostic findings, differential decision/ diagnoses, and management. (4) Provide guidance concerning the student's clinical progress, giving advice simultaneously on strengths and weaknesses (5) Plan additional learning experiences for the student (6) Verify the student's progress through written and oral evaluations (7) Share evaluations with the student and programme faculty.	The specific clinical experience developed in collaboration with a preceptor will vary depending on student objectives, the scope of the advanced role the student is preparing for and the country where the advanced nursing programme exists. Planned student experiences and related responsibilities can include the following under the supervision of or consultation with a preceptor (1) Set learning objectives (2) Obtain comprehensive health histories (3) Conduct physical examinations and related assessments (4) Order and interpret screening and diagnostic tests (5) Identify, evaluate and manage common acute, stable chronic or end-of-life conditions (6) Co-manage patients with complex health problems (7) Identify at risk factors and behaviors that influence health status (8) Evaluate emotional and social wellbeing (9) Develop health education and health promotion interventions (10) Collaborate with other health care professionals and make suitable referrals (11) Document findings in an organised, thorough manner (12) Evaluate clinical experience.

students. Illustrations describe the experience of physician preceptors in a community health clinical setting on the medical campus of Aga Khan University in Karachi, Pakistan and an NP clinical practicum coordinated with social services in Tai O on Lantau Island, China. The examples illustrate the collaborative efforts required to coordinate, teach and support students' clinical learning.

Students following the advanced clinical experience in Pakistan made the following comments:

Our role of counselling and teaching was very much appreciated.

Patients were receptive to being examined or advised by a nurse.

Doctors were learning from us and we learned from them. This will definitely impact nurses' image.

If we identified what was missed out, they [physicians] were appreciative rather than defensive.

One physician remarked: 'I am afraid if you set up a clinic next to me I will lose my patients to you.' (Gul, 2003)

Faculty background and preparation

In addressing the issue of faculty preparation for advanced practice at the master's level, the AACN (1996) recommends that faculty 'should have a strong theoretical and practice base in the field in which they teach' (p. 4). A widespread concern exists about the ability to launch and sustain new APN programmes given the scarcity of appropriately prepared faculty. The lack of faculty is a prob-

---

Vignette 5.4   Tai O community project: an innovative approach for nurse practitioner clinical practicum in Hong Kong.

One of the essential elements in APN and NP programmes is arranging and establishing clinical experiences. Finding actual practice settings can be problematic, especially in initial development. Hong Kong Polytechnic University School of Nursing NP Programme faced such a dilemma. The launching of the Tai O, Health Centre Project on Lantau Island provided one solution. The Rotary Club of Channel Islands granted funding to an established social services centre to offer rehabilitative services for the elderly suffering from stroke and associated debility of aging. This fishing village of 3500 people had 1000 identified elderly. Services were being organised under the direction of the Hong Kong Family Welfare Society. Tai O Jockey Club Clinic currently provides established medical and health care services.

A proposal from the Tai O social worker and service coordinator, Hong Kong Polytechnic University faculty, and NP students to include advanced clinical practicum was accepted. Presented as a pilot project, the NP students offered comprehensive examinations, clinical management and health education under direct supervision of an experienced NP. Referral patterns were established for pain management and rehabilitation with physiotherapists. Physician referral and backup was available at the Jockey Club Clinic. The Tai O Family Welfare office arranged appointments and resources.

The project provided students advanced clinical practicum in a community setting, introduced the NP role to other service providers while providing additional health care options to the elderly residents of the village. Continued student placement and plans to consider integrating an NP role into the service are positive outcomes of this project.

(M. Schober, personal communication)

Vignette 5.5 Developing advanced practice student clinical practicum on a medical campus in Pakistan.

At the Aga Khan University (AKU) in Karachi, Pakistan, the university has an established medical and nursing campus that includes outpatient health services. A masters in nursing with an APN focus was launched at Aga Khan University School of Nursing (AKUSON) in 2002. At the time faculty were exploring possibilities for student advanced clinical practicum experience, the idea of using physician preceptors in the outpatient clinic setting appeared to be a good option.

The concept of advanced nursing practice roles was known only to a select group of leaders at the school of nursing and medical school. The masters programme faculty had a variety of international educational experiences and the programme director from the United States had an NP background. Students in the programme were familiar with AKU medical staff as well as with the clinic services. Although cautious about the student placement from the outset, the director of clinic services and clinic physicians agreed to become clinical preceptors for the full-time students. Preceptor guidelines were provided and school of nursing faculty conducted site visits. Nursing students at times had clinical attachments along with medical students thus experiencing collaborative learning.

A challenge for faculty was to simultaneously explain the nature of the expected student learning experience to the preceptors, while ensuring course requirements were met. A cautious approach progressed to enthusiastic acceptance as students demonstrated their expertise and level of knowledge, and preceptors began to recognise and appreciate the value of nurses with advanced education. One of the students from the first group became a research collaborator with her physician preceptor.

(Y. Amarsi, personal communication; M. Schober site visit,
2002–2004)

---

lem even in countries with a long history in advanced nursing education, and may in the end be one of the most significant factors in limiting the dissemination of the role.

While educational institutions may have masters and doctoral prepared faculty or staff, this is no guarantee that they possess the necessary set of skills, knowledge and expertise to teach the theory and support clinical experience appropriate for advanced nursing practice. Strategies for faculty enhancement within the institution and for the continuing education of actual and potential faculty are critical to the long-term quality and sustainability of educational programmes. As interim measures institutions will probably draw on outside experts for help in the early stages of programme development and implementation until a critical mass of national faculty becomes available. (Doucette *et al.*, 2005, key informants, personal communication).

As faculty have a fundamental responsibility for guiding, supervising and evaluating student practice, maintaining currency in clinical practice is another area to confront. Recognition of this requirement is important and institutions have a responsibility to assist faculty to achieve this goal (NTF, 2002). Including a clinical practice element as part of formal faculty job requirements is advised. In turn, faculty will be required to provide periodic evidence of practice arrangements and experience.

Professional development and continuing education

Continuing education (CE) and professional development following completion of an educational programme are viewed as necessary to maintain and continue to refine skills and knowledge. There is a perception that appropriate continuing education for advanced practice is a way to assure the quality of health care service provision. In some countries the maintenance of a credentialed status for advanced practice is tied to completion of specified continuing education requirements (Hanson, 2005; key informants, personal communication). Nurse practitioners who were interviewed in Australia and New Zealand recognised that knowledge for sound practice requires individual effort to consistently update 'currency of clinical knowledge' (Gardner *et al.*, 2004, p. 45). Information introducing strategies for nursing and midwifery workforce enhancement in Southeast Asia emphasises the value of continuing education to strengthen competency based education and life-long learning (WHO-SEARO, 2003).

A study done by Andersson (2001) at the Department of Advanced Nursing Education at Goteborg University, Sweden, concluded that CE contributes to positive development at the level of personal knowledge and capability. However, CE does not necessarily lead to changes in work situations or benefits in terms of compensation or professional recognition. In spite of the attainment of professional goals and enhanced self-confidence, respondents in this study voiced an expectation that undertaking CE should be associated with improved pay, practice options and influence in the work setting.

While support and interest in concepts such as life-long learning and other CE benefits is voiced, responses from key informants fail to support CE as a universal requirement for advanced nursing practice. Additionally, in countries where respondents report CE to be recommended or mandatory, criteria are varied and inconsistent. It appears the value of CE and its place in advanced nursing practice as related to professional competence requires further exploration and research.

In initial discussion, the ICN INP/APNN Network (ICN, 2005) suggests the following professional development competencies for APNs. The APN:

(1) Carries out regular review of own practice through peer review and other mechanisms
(2) Contributes to new knowledge and practice development by maintaining currency of scientific and technological advancements in nursing
(3) Evaluates health outcomes of advanced practice services to assist in shaping care and nursing practice

(4) Participates in local and national policy-making, in concert with professional organisations, to influence equitable health care and the maintenance of the NP/APN role

(5) Provides leadership among peers in formulating and implementing policies, standards and procedures for advanced practice in the work environment

(6) Is organised professionally to promote the APN role through the refinement of measurable competency criteria that contribute to improve health care.

Educational standards and programme accreditation

The National Task Force on Quality Nurse Practitioner Education (2002) provides a standard framework to be used in the review of NP programmes in the United States in order to ensure currency, relevancy and quality of NP education in the country. A wide spectrum of stakeholders (faculty, administrators, students, accrediting and certifying organisations, and consumers) contributed to the standards cited in the document. The criteria are meant to provide guidance in six programme development areas: organisation and administration, students, faculty, curriculum, resources and evaluation. Use of information from this document and other sources from the United States appear to be significant because as advanced nursing practice progresses internationally, the authors acknowledge that patterns of educational programmes adopted at country level are often inspired by, and a reflection of, some aspect of what has happened in the United States (Gardner *et al.*, 2004; Hong Kong Polytechnic University School of Nursing, 2004; NCNZ, 2002; NHI Botswana, 1986; RCN, 2002; key informants, personal communication). The authors acknowledge that further study is needed to evaluate the impact that this influence has on APN programme development globally.

Accreditation as it relates to educational programmes is further discussed in Chapter 4.

Conclusion

Sound educational programmes are essential for promoting the APN as a credible and accepted member of the global health workforce. This chapter has emphasised the necessity to offer education consistent with a defined advanced nursing scope of practice, which at the same time reflects the needs of the population and related health care services. A flexible framework for curriculum development is suggested and the diversity of educational initiatives under way is illustrated through real-life examples. Finally guidelines for designing and establishing clinical experiences and preceptor relationships have been presented.

The authors hope that with time, further research and consensus on internationally agreed definitions of the scope of practice will provide a more precise picture of what trends and commonalities are important in advanced nursing practice education. Of further interest would be to assess the influence and impact the dominance of one country on the development of advanced nursing globally. Scrutiny of what succeeded and what failed when adapting existing models and educational programmes for a new context will be most useful in providing practical educational guidelines for those facing this task.

As interest in advanced nursing practice continues and as the diversity of practice and educational approaches grow, the authors look forward to a growth in the body of experiential knowledge and research data that will continue to provide an evidence base to guide and improve educational strategies.

References

American Association of Colleges of Nursing. (2004). *Position statement on the practice doctorate in nursing.* Washington D. C.: Author.

American Association of Colleges of Nursing. (1996). *The Essentials of master's education for advanced practice nursing.* Washington, D.C.: Author.

An Bord Altranis. (2003). *Guidelines on the key points that may be considered when developing a quality clinical learning environment,* 1st Edition. Dublin: Author.

Andersson, E.P. (2001). Continuing education in Sweden – to what purpose? *Journal of Continuing Education in Nursing,* **32**(2) 86–93.

Aga Khan University School of Nursing. (2004). *Master of Science in nursing programme documents.* Karachi: Author.

Canadian Nurses Association. (2002). *Advanced nursing practice: A national framework.* Revised. Ottawa: Author.

Canadian Nurse Practitioner Initiative. (CNPI) (2004). *Canadian nurse practitioner initiative develops Pan-Canadian framework for the sustained integration of nurse practitioners.* Information series. Ottawa: Author.

Canadian Nurses Association. (2004). *Achieving excellence in professional practice. A guide to preceptorship and mentorship.* Ottawa: Author.

Castledine, G. (2003). The development of advanced practice nursing practice in the UK. In P. McGee, G. Castledine (Eds) *Advanced nursing practice,* 2nd Edition, pp. 8–16. Oxford: Blackwell Publishing.

Castledine, G. (2005). *Ensuring competence of the advanced practice nurse.* Conference workshop for the conference Advanced Nursing Practice: Moving Forward, Singapore.

Dahlgren, G., Whitehead, M. (1991). *Policies and strategies to promote social equity in health.* Stockholm: Institute for Fiscal Affairs.

Doucette, S., Duff, E., Sangster-Gormley, E. (2005). *Nurse practitioner education in Canada: transforming the future.* Presented at the National Organization of Nurse Practitioner Faculties annual conference. Retrieved August 28, 2005 from http://www.icn-apnetwork.org

Gagan, M.J., Berg, J., Root, S. (2002). Nurse practitioner curriculum for the 21st century: a model for evaluation and revision. *Journal of Nursing Education,* **41**(5), pp. 2002–2006.

Gardner, G., Carryer, J., Dunn, S., Gardner, A. (2004). *Nurse Practitioner Standards Project.* Report to the Australian Nursing Council: Author.

Gul, R. (2003). Focusing on APN through a graduate programme. Presented at ICN Conference. Geneva, Switzerland. Retrieved October 24, 2005 from http://www.icn-apnetwork.org

Hanson, C.M. (2005). Understanding regulatory, legal, and credentialing requirements. In A.B. Hamric, J.A. Spross, C.M. Hanson (Eds) *Advanced practice nursing: An integrative approach,* 3rd Edition, pp. 781–808. St. Louis: Elsevier Saunders.

Hong Kong Polytechnic University School of Nursing. (2004). *Definitive programme document: Master of Science in Nursing*. Hong Kong: Author.

Inman, C. (2003). Providing a culture of learning for advanced practice students undertaking a master's degree. In P. McGee, G. Castledine (2003) *Advanced nursing practice*, 2nd Edition, pp. 73–84. Oxford: Blackwell Publishing.

International Council of Nurses. (2002). *Definition and characteristics of the role*. Retrieved August 30, 2005 from http://www.icn-apnetwork.org

International Council of Nurses. (2005). *The scope of practice, standards and competencies of the advanced practice nurse*. Working Draft. Geneva: Author. Retrieved August 30, 2005 from http://www.icn-apnetwork.org

Maclaine, K., Walsh, M., Harston, B. (2004). *Embracing nurse practitioners within the post-registration regulatory framework*. Paper submitted for Post-Registration Review Conference. Royal College of Nursing: Unpublished.

McKenna H., Cutcliffe, J. (2001). Doctoral education in the United Kingdom and Ireland. *Online Journal of Issues in Nursing*. Vol. 5, No. 2. Retrieved December 27, 2005 from http://www.nursingworld.org/ojin/topic12/tpc12_9.htm

National Health Institute. (1986). *Curriculum for training of the family nurse practitioners: post basic course*. Gaborone: Author.

National Organization of Nurse Practitioner Faculties (NONPF). (1995). *Advanced nursing practice: curriculum guidelines and program standards for nurse practitioner education*. Washington, D.C.: Author.

National Organization of Nurse Practitioner Faculties (NONPF). (2000). *Domains and competencies of nurse practitioner practice*. Washington DC: author.

National Task Force on Quality Nurse Practitioner Education (NTF). (2002). *Criteria for evaluation of nurse practitioner programs*. Washington, D.C.: Author.

National University of Singapore. (2005). Academic preparation for advanced practice nurses in Singapore. Presented at the International Nursing Conference sponsored by the National University of Singapore entitled 'Advanced Nursing Practice: Moving Forward'. Retrieved March 14, 2006 from http://www.nuh.com.sg/apn2005/apn2005_handouts.htm

Nursing Council of New Zealand (NCNZ). (2002). *The nurse practitioner: responding to health needs in New Zealand*. NCNZ: Author.

Nurses and Midwives Board of New South Wales. (2005). *Nurse practitioner authorization*. Retrieved September 23, 2005 from nursesreg.nsw.gov.au/np_options.htm

O'Malley, C., Cunliffe, E., Hunter, S., Breeze., J. (2000). Preceptorship in practice. *Nursing Standard*, **14**(28), 45–49.

Royal College of Nursing. (2002, Revised 2005). *Nurse practitioners – an RCN guide to the nurse practitioner role, competencies and programme approval*. London: Author.

Schober, M., McKay, N. (2004). *Collaborative practice in the 21st Century*. [Monograph]. Geneva: International Council of Nurses.

Seitio, O.S. (2000). *The family nurse practitioner in Botswana: issues and challenges*. Presented at the 8th International NP Conference, San Diego, California.

Skills for Health. (2005). *Key elements for a career framework*. Retrieved 27 December, 2005 from http://www.skillsforhealth.org.uk/careerframework/key_elements.php

Spross, J.A. (2005). Expert coaching and guidance. In A.B. Hamric, J.A. Spross, C.M. Hanson (Eds) *Advanced practice nursing: An integrative approach*, 3rd Edition, pp. 187–223. St. Louis: Elsevier Saunders.

State Government of Victoria, Australia, Department of Human Services. (2005). *Nursing in Victoria: Nurse practitioner*. Retrieved September 25, 2005 http:www.nursing.vic.gov.au/furthering/practitioner.htm

Styles, M.M., Affara F.A. (1997). *ICN on regulation: Towards a 21st century model*. Geneva: International Council of Nurses.

Taylor-Seehafer, M.A., Abel, E., Tyler, D.O., Sonstein, F.C. (2004). Integrating evidence-based practice in nurse practitioner education. *Journal of the American Academy of Nurse Practitioners*, **16**(12), 520–525.

Towers, J. (January 2005). After forty years. *Journal of the American Academy of Nurse Practitioners*, **17**(1), 9–13.

University of Skovde. (2003). *Advanced nursing practice in primary health care study programme*. Skovde, Sweden. Retrieved June 7, 2005 from www.icn-apnetwork.org

University of South Carolina. *Family and community health, nurse practitioner preceptor guidelines*. Retrieved June 7, 2005 from www.sc.edu/nursing/npguideprecept.html

University of Stirling. (Undated). *Doctor of nursing. Doctor of midwifery*. Stirling: Author. Retrieved December 27, 2005 from http://www.nm.stir.ac.uk/postgrad/intro.htm

World Health Organization. (2005). WHO supports integrative management of childhood illness and advanced practice nurse training in Timor-Leste. *Public Information and Events*, **3**(2). Retrieved June 21, 2005 from w3.whosea.org/LinkFiles/Public_Information_&_Events_vol3-2_timor-leste.pdf

World Health Organization-South-East Asia. (2003). *Nursing and midwifery workforce management: Conceptual framework*. SEARO Technical Publication, No. 25. New Delhi: Author.

World Health Organization-Western Pacific Region (WHO-WPRO). (2001). *Mid-level and nurse practitioners in the Pacific: models and issues*. Manila: Author.

Chapter 6
Research

Theoretical perspective of advanced nursing practice

> Is there evidence of a theoretical foundation unique to advanced nursing practice?
>
> What specific body of knowledge drives advanced practice?

Nicoteri and Andrews (2003) explored these questions in relation to nurse practitioners (NP) suggesting that if a specific body of knowledge could be identified that is unique to NP practice, educators would have a solid foundation for teaching students, and researchers would have a paradigm to use in investigating advanced nursing practice and related issues. After reviewing literature from the United States and Canada these authors concluded that, although the NP role evolved from nursing, it is heavily influenced by medicine. There was evidence from this review that the emergent theories specific to NPs have theoretical starting points originating in nursing, medicine and social science. Analysis of early NP research done by Hughes *et al.* (2003) concluded that the studies were carried out to legitimatise and provide support for these new nursing services, but lacked a sound theoretical approach.

In addressing the importance of using a conceptual model of nursing as a guide for advanced practice roles, Fawcett *et al.* (2004) suggest that advanced roles are built on the caring nature of nursing. Hagedorn and Quinn (2004) describe and also attempt to support the perspective that caring theory guides NP practice. While acknowledging that in the past theory-based practice concentrated on conceptual models of nursing to guide care, Brown (2005) suggests that the emphasis has shifted to middle-range theories[1] that more specifically guide advanced practice.

Following a literature review, Woods (2000) writes that operational and conceptual models for advanced nursing practice are evolving. It appears that historical models, in general, rest on identification of defining tasks and behaviours for advanced practice. This has resulted in operational models based on attempts to put forward abstract constructs or conceptual frameworks. This author focuses on the two dominant operational models of the NP and the clinical nurse specialist (CNS). In using this approach, Woods emphasises models that describe attributes and characteristics associated with advanced practice, and that are developed to a level of expertise that differentiates advanced from generalist nursing.

The theoretical basis of nursing has become a core topic in the education of professional nurses (Nicoteri & Andrews, 2003). Theory as it relates to nursing practice is often included in baccalaureate education. Varying levels of emphasis on theory and theory development are provided in graduate education, including programmes designed for advanced nursing practice. Integral to this trend is a view that theory determines what is meaningful as a result of study, exploration and the presentation of evidence (Fawcett *et al.*, 2001). According to Brown (2005) APNs are becoming comfortable with the idea of evidence-based practice, yet the idea of theory-based practice is less familiar to them. Theory can be a very practical tool that 'often brings together research findings in a way that helps practice be more purposeful, systematic, and comprehensive' (p. 163). The challenge seems to lie in connecting the theory to clinical practice.

As key stakeholders require more evidence to be convinced as to the benefits that advanced nursing practice brings to improving health care, more research is needed to articulate a body of knowledge clearly associated with advanced nursing practice. As a result there is increased interest in identifying theories and conceptual models relevant for advanced practice.

McGee and Castledine (2003) point out that '*advanced practice is a state of professional maturity*' in which the '*advanced practitioner is able to draw on scholarly, interpersonal and reflective skills*' (p. 226). Comments from key informants (personal communication) indicate that there is interest in developing theoretical frameworks or conceptual models that could embrace all areas of practice

---

[1] A middle-range theory encompasses a limited scope with a limited number of variables that are testable in a direct manner.

while providing a foundation to promote uniformity, continuity and agreement on the core principles of advanced practice.

Exploring the research perspective

Why is it important for advanced practice nurses to integrate scholarly expertise and knowledge of research activities into advanced practice?

The scope of practice and the characteristics of expanded clinical nursing are worthy of inquiry and clarification if it is to secure its place in what are increasingly dynamic health care environments. There is value in discovering the impact of the presence of APNs on health policy, health care outcomes and health care systems worldwide. Usable models and frameworks for practice are beneficial as global interest in the use of advanced nursing skills heightens. Key informants support this view and emphasise the need for international assistance from organisations such as the International Council of Nurses to promote and pursue a research agenda that focuses on these themes.

In order to explore as well as pursue a research agenda for advanced practice, nurses need to acquire knowledge and skills necessary for research competence. Research questions requiring effective study are often related to best practice for a specific patient population; identification of factors that affect outcomes in a variety of health problems; and indicators of quality care in advanced practice (Hickey, 2000). In addressing the subject of skills-mix in provision of health care along with reviewing the evidence that supports the expansion of nursing services, Buchan and Dal Poz (2002) observe that more extensive and diverse research and improved methodologies would add strength to the currently available body of literature representing advanced nursing practice.

Gardner *et al.* (2004) suggest increased utilisation of mixed methods of research to provide prospective population-based epidemiological data to more accurately assess outcomes, cost-effectiveness and the occurrence of advanced nursing services. Additionally, these researchers advocate that research focus on evaluation of patient outcomes, interdisciplinary professional efforts, and scope of practice. In describing the rationale for scholarly inquiry and future directions in advanced nursing practice, McGee and Castledine (2003) emphasise the 'need for new emergent nursing roles to retain their professional identity and avoid over reliance on the medical model or its associated technology' (p. 225). This will enable advanced nursing practice to continue to establish its own body of knowledge.

Key informants confirm the importance of research and inquiry related to advanced nursing roles; however, recommendations for what to investigate vary in theme and topic. Furthermore, to have a broader global perspective, data and descriptions are needed from areas of the world where advanced nursing activities occur, but are currently under-represented or not represented at all in publications. This makes it all the more important that as advanced nursing pro-grammes develop internationally, research skills and competencies become an integral part of the role. A more in-depth discussion on enhancing knowledge and skills in research and a research agenda for advanced nursing practice is found later in this chapter.

Promoting diverse and analytical research

In reviewing international literature associated with various advanced practice roles Buchan & Dal Poz (2002), Gardner *et al.* (2004), and Hughes *et al.* (2003) agree that the majority of papers consist of editorials, anecdotal descriptions and commentaries on practice models or illustrations of curriculum design. In assessing the significance of this research and data it is further noted that a sub-stantial number of published studies are mainly narrative accounts, while other studies have methodological limitations. Additionally, most analytical studies have been conducted in the United States although there are noteworthy con-tributions from Canada and the United Kingdom with the beginning emergence of publications from Australia, New Zealand and Southeast Asia (Buchan & Calman, 2004; key informants, personal communication). Refer to the biblio-graphy for publications and research articles as provided by key informants.

Based on the currently available body of research, reports and analyses, a case can be made that introducing APNs into the health workforce contributes to maintaining and improving quality of care. There is evidence that the strategy of increasing the utilisation of nurses within expanded roles has the potential to contribute to cost-effectiveness and cost containment in provision of com-prehensive health care. However, while recognising that limitations to change may exist, further studies are needed to clarify the boundaries for advanced nurs-ing practice, and the relationship with other health professionals, especially physi-cians, that are most favourable to good practice. No research has addressed this clearly, and the current standards associated with advanced nursing practice do not appear to be based on research findings (Buchan & Calman, 2004; Gardner *et al.* 2004, key informants, personal communication).

Research for advocacy

Increasingly data from credible research are required to support the case for change or innovation. It is therefore important to be aware of factors that promote or hinder the use of data and research in advocacy work and policy development (Sharma, undated). Brehaut and Juzwishin (2005) write that the failure to take up even high-quality research evidence by decision-makers has been called the 'gap between research and policy. The research community has devoted much time and energy to talking about bridging the gap between research and decision-making, but today significant chasms still exist between

Table 6.1 Factors that hinder or promote use of data and research. (Source: Adapted from Sharma, undated, p. 20.)

Factors which *promote* use of data and research	Factors which *hinder* the use of data and research
Design the study taking into account the information needs of key stakeholders.	Research studies and findings that are not relevant to policy decisions.
Policy makers should perceive the research as credible and reliable.	Timing is off: research findings answer questions that are no longer of interest or needed.
Focus research on a few questions that can be answered.	Presentation or conduct by researcher(s) not credible to the key stakeholders.
Present findings in multiple formats tailored to the audience.	
Disseminate findings using a variety of methods while also ensuring that the same information is conveyed to everyone.	Findings are inconclusive or subject to widely different interpretations.
	Findings are not generalisable.
Emphasise the importance of the findings rather than the need for more research.	Reported findings are lengthy, too technical or plagued by excess jargon.
	Findings are not widely distributed.

the two' (p. 6). Stocking (1995, as cited in Brehaut & Juzwishin, 2005), provides commentary on why research findings are not used and identifies the following four reasons:

● The research is not there.
● Many decision-makers are not knowledgeable or may not have the ability to interpret the information.
● Public health (and others) does not act as an advocate of knowledge.
● Change is more difficult than expected.

Refer to Table 6.1 for suggestions that will help ensure that information and evidence adds to the body of advanced nursing practice knowledge, as well being usable for advocacy work.

Enhancing knowledge and skills in research

What factors influence interest in contributing to advanced nursing research?

What knowledge or skills would promote participation of APNs in research activities?

- Facilitation, support and encouragement
- Role modeling
- Consistency in determining relevance to practice
- Identified applications for clinical practice

Figure 6.1   Strategies to increase research awareness. (Source: Camiah, 1997.)

The research culture

Through structured inquiry, research provides knowledge to enhance understanding as well as promote the development and implementation of advanced
nursing practice. Descriptions and definitions of advanced practice often include
research as a professional-role activity. However, a combination of factors
appears to contribute to almost a disconnect between nursing and comfort with
the research process. Reasons proposed for this include: lack of awareness and
interest in research literature; absence of encouragement or motivation to apply
research findings; poor access to research literature; inapplicable research findings; and nurses who are not educated in the benefits and understanding of
research (Champion & Leach, 1989; Closs and Cheater, 1994; Holzemer, 1998).
Too often nurses are not proficient in reading research literature. All these factors
inhibit a positive perception on the part of nurses to do research, and limit use
of research findings and involvement in research projects.

May *et al.* (1998), believing that there are certain attributes of context or
culture that can increase awareness and participation in research, studied the
way nurses think about it, the value placed on research and its relevance to practice. Recommendations from this study propose strategies to reduce fears and
misperceptions associated with research. These include understanding research
application to practice, greater knowledge of the complexities of the research
process, methodical education in research skills, and finding ways to identify
research needs relevant to work settings. Consistent with this view are study findings
by Camiah (1997) who suggests four strategies to increase research awareness
for students and qualified nurses and promote a more positive research culture
in nursing (Figure 6.1).

It appears that a positive research culture is advantageous for promotion of
nursing research utilisation and investigation. When research competence is perceived to be a valued and rewarded activity, interested parties and key stakeholders will have improved access to an expanding body of knowledge on which
to base decision-making.

Research competence

In describing research competence De Palma and McGuire (2005) name three
research competencies viewed as necessary for advanced practice nurses (Figure 6.2). Similarly, the research role of the advanced practice nurse is described
by Kraus (2000) as including research utilisation or application to practice and

- Interpretation and use of research
- Evaluation of practice
- Participation in collaborative research

Figure 6.2 Research competencies. (Source: DePalma & McGuire, 2005, p. 295.)

the conduct of research. Understanding the research process and steps to take in project development facilitates action toward rigorous participation. See Figure 6.3 for a depiction of this process. Advanced practice nurses with varying levels of research competence have the potential of contributing to documenting and validating the strengths or limitations of advanced clinical practice.

Diverse research that contributes to understanding of quality outcomes for advanced practice will assist APNs to articulate aspects of their services that make a difference to the health of populations. Acknowledgement that APNs need research skills to provide quality health care, initiate change and improve nursing practice is consistent with the move towards higher levels of education (American Association of Colleges of Nursing [AACN], 1996; American Nurses Association [ANA], 1996). Introduction of research courses in the curriculum prepares a professional capable of evaluating research; has the capacity to identify problems for investigation in clinical practice; asks research questions; and is aware of practice outcomes and clinical applications of research findings. One dilemma that the APN is likely to face is how to fit research related activities into a schedule of complex and intense practice responsibilities (Kraus, 2000).

Writing for publication

Additions to the body of advanced practice literature and publications are dependent on the ability of the APN to communicate research findings and describe practice settings through writing. The skill of developing and writing about a theme or topic for the purpose of publication promotes clinical thinking and clinical judgement useful for data analysis and problem solving.

De Back (2005) encourages nurses to move from personal descriptive stories to scholarly writing that is based on and demonstrates outcomes or benefits achieved from restructuring of systems. Publication of findings of a scholarly nature based on systematically collected information contributes to knowledge and documentation on advanced practice. Even more importantly, in the current dynamic environment, advanced practice nurses need to write and share information so that others have access to it.

Starting to write

Inherent to the expectation that APNs write about their practice, is the degree of confidence with which an individual is able to approach the point where

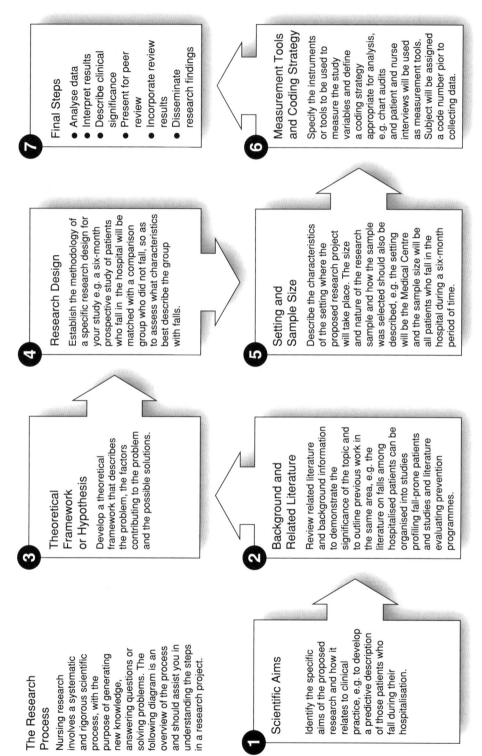

Figure 6.3   The research process. (Source ICN, retrieved 2005, from http://www.icn.ch/resnet.htm)

- Is the subject material or topic original?
- Does the information build on work by others?
- What is it about the idea or approach that offers good reason for publication?
- What is the significance or relevance of the report, story or research?
- How will the publication contribute to or improve knowledge or practice?
- Does the work or results have widespread application?
- Will inclusion of a co-author strengthen the manuscript?
- What are the most important aspects of the work that should be included in the manuscript?

Figure 6.4 Preparing to write. (Source: De Back, 2001.)

writing starts. In the development of writing skills the first step is to make a decision about a topic or theme for possible publication. Writing begins with thinking about the topic to be described. This is followed by the translation of complex thinking into clear language. In the International Council of Nurses (ICN) manual for authors, De Back (2005) offers suggestions of questions to ask when preparing or planning to write (Figure 6.4).

Writing

After the 'thinking' process, the next step is to develop an objective to guide the writing process. Having a clear and simple written objective provides focus for the text. For example: Describe the impact of advanced practice nurse prescribing on primary health care service delivery in rural areas of China. Ask what the reader will gain, know or understand after reading the text or article?

The next stage is to develop an outline or structural design to guide the writing process. Develop a style that is natural. Consider starting with the conclusion or stated objective of the project in order to achieve content that is consistent with the stated endpoint (Figure 6.5).

In the beginning of writing, concentrate on content rather than manner of writing, and continue to write steadily. Refinement of style and subject matter will occur in the revision process. Figure 6.6 gives some hints to help you adopt a clear, fluent writing style.

- Introduction
- Definition of topic or theme
- Description of scope of the article
- Documentation of prior work on the topic
- Significance or relevance of the information
- Clearly describe data, collective information and useful application
- Identify tables or figures
- Conclusion

Figure 6.5 Guidelines for preparing an outline for writing. (Source: De Back, 2001.)

- Writing style is distinctive to the author. Develop your own approach.
- Write as simply as possible using short words, short sentences and short paragraphs.
- Write clearly. Avoid slang or terminology that is not universal.
- Specific terms are preferable to vague terminology.
- Focus on the central message of the manuscript.
- Continue writing.

Figure 6.6   Hints for writing. (Source: De Back, 2001.)

Manuscript preparation

In manuscript preparation, following author guidelines for a specific journal as well as use of a writing checklist will ensure that a manuscript is in an appropriate format for submission to a journal or publication editor. See Appendix 7 for an example checklist for authors in submitting a manuscript for peer review and refer to http://www.icn.ch/inr.htm for an example of guidelines for authors for the ICN journal *International Nursing Review*.

As professionals and innovators, advanced practice nurses are expected to develop research and writing skills in order to advance the profession through dissemination of descriptions of innovation in clinical practice and outcomes studies. Writing and publishing enhances the communication of observations and data thus contributing to an increased body of knowledge. The authors hope that the suggestions provided will encourage the novice as well the more experienced writer to record and publish evidence as well as the experiences of advanced nursing practice.

Searching for research funding

Key informants (personal communication) emphasise the need for collaborative international research on advanced nursing practice as this collective knowledge will add to the comprehension of the various facets of these new nursing roles. Funding sources are essential for maintenance of a research infrastructure that allows identification of research needs, the conduct of research and dissemination of findings. Historically in many countries, funding sources have supported medical research and nursing has had limited access to these funds. Persuading funding agencies to support nursing research for advanced practice will require collective action of researchers, educational institutions, professional associations and governmental authorities. Allocation of funding will rest on sound proposals, organised, pertinent research goals, and priorities (Holzemer, 1998). Strategies to identify financial support from public and private sectors will help to move a research agenda forward; therefore this task should not be neglected.

In an advocacy-training guide for fundraising, Sharma (undated) describes the diversity of funding sources that should be explored when fund raising for research

- Individuals
- Private sector companies (including multinationals)
- Philanthropic/donor agencies and foundations
- Government sponsored initiatives
- Academic resources

Figure 6.7   Funding sources. (Source: Sharma, undated.)

(Figure 6.7). It is important to match the theme of the proposal or project to the funder(s) most likely to be interested in the study or project. Potential funders may have restrictions or specific conditions attached to the kind of initiatives they are likely to support. Certain conditions might conflict with the type of research activity proposed. Laws in certain countries govern financial support for projects. Plan to become informed of these issues in order to develop a proposal more likely to obtain a positive response from funders.

Specific actions taken by the researcher can increase the likelihood of obtaining financial support:

- Clearly describe what distinguishes this research proposal from others in the field.
- Define the reasons why this work could benefit advanced nursing practice.
- Realistically assess the likelihood that a potential donor would be interested in the research.
- Investigate multiple sources to diversify the funding base.
- Develop a budget.
- Provide background and information to support the credibility of the researcher(s).

If a research proposal has been rejected for funding determine why and evaluate if there are acceptable changes that could be made to ensure future financial support. Once funding has been provided for the research proposal, maintain good fiscal management, keep funding sources informed and up to date on the progress and action timelines of the work being done.

International Classification for Nursing Practice® (ICNP): a tool for collaborative nursing research

As far back as the late 1980s, the membership of ICN recognised the need for a unified nursing language to describe the patient phenomenon of concern to nursing. In the introduction to Version 1 of the International Classification for Nursing Practice® (ICNP), ICN observed that what nurses need is a shared terminology to 'express the elements of nursing practice (what nurses do, relative to certain human needs or patient conditions, to produce certain outcomes)' (ICN, 2005a, p. 7).

Prime movers behind the search for a unified language for nursing were the increasing use of electronic health records and computer-based information systems in clinical settings, and a growing need for technology to support evidence based practice. Also with the globalisation of health, the issue of communication at international levels was brought sharply into focus; the task is made difficult as multiple nursing terminologies have grown around its many specialties and subspecialties.

The purpose of ICNP® is to provide a unifying framework 'to bring together nursing practice data from across the world and to incorporate this data into its nursing information system' (ICN, 2005a, p. 27) To accomplish this, ICNP® developers created a structure capable of making nursing data used in health systems worldwide readily available. Version 1 through its unifying structure allows nurses to cross-map local, natural language to a standard meaning.

Version 1 of the ICNP® was launched in May 2005. The foreword notes that it is a dynamic and progressive tool which has the following benefits:

- It establishes a common language for describing nursing practice in order to improve communication among nurses and between nurses and others.
- It represents concepts used in local practice, across languages and specialty areas.
- It describes the nursing care of people (individuals, families and communities) worldwide.
- It enables comparison of nursing data across client populations, settings, geographical areas and time.
- It stimulates nursing research through links to data available in nursing and health information systems.
- It provides data about nursing practice in order to influence decision-making, education and health policy.
- It projects trends in patient needs, provision of nursing care, resource utilisation and outcomes of nursing care.

As nursing knowledge is continually extended through research and development, the ICNP® will strive to continually represent nursing in all its depth and breadth. It is hoped that the focus on clinical research stimulated by the growth and growing confidence of advanced nursing practice will enable APNs to become a major source of well-documented research on terminology describing their practice, and which will eventually feed into the ICNP®. To aid with this research task, ICN has set up accredited centres for ICNP® research and development. This can be an institution, faculty, department, national association or other group meeting ICN criteria or groups that extend across countries and regions. The ICNP® centre may be organised by language, by specialisation or by research expertise. A list of ICN accredited centres is available in resources section.

The ICNP® developers understood that nurses needed relevant sets of pre-coordinated statements of nursing diagnoses, interventions and outcome statements to ease documentation. With the release of version 1 of the ICNP®, work will begin on catalogues which are subsets of nursing diagnoses, interventions and outcomes for a selected area or sub-specialty. This presents opportunities for advanced nursing practice researchers to examine their specialist area of practice from the point of view of what exists in the ICNP®, identify what is lacking, and begin to:

- Develop a catalogue specific to a specific area of practice. See Appendix 8 for an example of a catalogue.
- Submit terms to the CNP® to be considered for the next version of the ICNP®.

The reader is referred to the ICNP® web page (http://www.icn.ch/icnp_review.htm) for more information on how to submit terms.

An international research agenda for advanced nursing practice

> In developing an international research agenda for advanced nursing practice, what is it that key stakeholders want to know?
>
> What areas of study would contribute to a greater understanding and development of advanced nursing within the international context?
>
> How do these concepts and themes specifically translate into a research agenda for the advancement of nursing?
>
> Does current research accurately reflect the reality of clinical practice worldwide?

From an international perspective numerous limitations arise with any publication, analyses of literature reviews, or organisational reports. Most publications are written in English eliminating access to the non-English speaker, and limiting comprehension to those whose primary language is not English. Publications unavailable in English are inaccessible to the broader international audience unless they are translated into either English or another language thus limiting accessibility and wider dissemination. An English speaker lacks access to conceptual material on emerging roles as a result of unfamiliarity with regional or country specific languages or dialects.

Hughes *et al.* (2003) comment that key stakeholders inquiring into advanced practice in countries outside of the United States experience frustration in evaluating adaptability of advanced practice characteristics and concepts to settings where the scope of practice, practice settings and health systems are very different. Added to this is the grey literature representing a wealth of national and local experiences that are inaccessible, difficult to acquire or locate, or are available only in a non-transmittable form. It would seem that accessible data provide a limited and biased view of the realities and potential of advanced clinical practice within the global context.

In presenting key questions for a research agenda McGee and Castledine (2003) suggest nine themes for inquiry into the issues and realities of implementing advanced nursing practice roles. These recommended themes are 'clinical practice', 'evidence-based practice', 'diversity and inclusiveness', 'interface with other service providers', 'professional regulations and control', 'providing professional leadership', 'user view', 'education' and 'recording of historical developments' (pp. 227–232). Research themes for a research agenda place a strong concentration on clinical practice issues, while recognising the need to take into account topics related to health policy and multidisciplinary collaboration. De Palma and McGuire (2005) support the view that research is essential as advanced practice nurses *'define, implement, refine, validate, and evaluate their practices'* (p. 295).

The key informants (personal communication) elicited a rich list of recommendations for an international research agenda. Figure 6.8 presents the responses organised according to McGee and Castledine's (2003) defined areas for APN research. The topics form broad areas for formulating pertinent research questions.

Recommendations for a research agenda emphasised the need for more diverse and inclusive studies demonstrating patient outcomes that are associated with the effectiveness and quality of services provided by APNs. Furthermore, comments stressed that, although there is interest in comparing advanced nursing practice to medical practice outcomes, research needs to move beyond these comparisons to studying outcomes directly related to advanced nursing practice. For example: What is achieved by health services provided by advanced practice nurses? What are the parameters of service design and delivery that support positive outcomes? Overall a consensus emerged to promote a research platform for increased collaboration and conduct of studies among countries to better understand the multiplicity of issues identified in the proposed advanced nursing research agenda.

The future research agenda related to advanced practice is multifaceted, extensive and diverse in this dynamic and ever changing field of nursing. The authors strongly advocate identification of research priorities that provide a focus on issues that are urgently needed to provide conceptual clarity for all stakeholders as well as nurses investigating these new roles. Of utmost importance is the challenge to proceed with rigorous methodology and consistent terminology to identify models and frameworks that are usable and adaptable in defining who an advanced practice nurse is and what advanced nursing practice is. Improved empirical understanding, consensus on role boundaries and interaction with other disciplines, policy makers and the public would appear to ensure a better understanding of the value these nurses bring to multiple dimensions of health care. Included in this vital topic is the necessity to identify career frameworks that not only describe characteristics and competencies associated with advanced practice but clinical pathways that are rewarding and appealing.

An additional area the authors believe requires the immediate attention of researchers is more extensive and rigorous study evaluating clinical outcomes related to not only the presence of all APN roles but value and impact on patient outcomes. This priority was most frequently named by key informants (personal communication) as information needed to move the advanced nursing practice

Clinical practice
Clinical outcomes for APN
Satisfaction and acceptance of patients, employers, other health professionals and nursing colleagues
Determinants of practice and role development: novice to expert
Best practice models
Cost effectiveness and funding
Fees/reimbursement/salaries commensurate with service provision
Practice guidelines
Relevant practice settings
Role support

Evidenced based practice (based also on ability to evaluate the evidence)
Studies demonstrating direct benefits to specific populations
Targeted outcomes related to specific disease categories
Effective health promotion & illness prevention outcomes
Quality and safety of care issues

Diversity and inclusiveness
Appropriate cultural approaches for diverse populations seeking care
Providing appropriate health care services according to specific population needs

Interface with other professionals
Impact of advanced nursing practice on other health care providers
Benefits and strategies of collaboration and health care teams
Effective strategies to overcome obstacles with other professionals

Standards and regulation
Approaches to defining and demonstrating competence
Effective methods for establishing scope of practice, standards, regulation, legislation
Relevance of standards
Evaluation of incentive schemes and career ladders
Legal implications/indemnity insurance

Professional leadership
Examples and traits of sound effectual transformational leadership
Effective behaviours of leadership
Nurse-led and managed service models
Human resource planning in the face of workforce shortages

User/consumer view
Delivering service identified by public needs
Pinpointing views and beliefs of those seeking services
Understanding user concerns and where they get their information

Education
Appraisals of advanced practice education curriculum requirements
Evaluations of the adequacy of role preparation
Qualities of effective educators
Continuing education
Continuing professional competence

Historical development
Maintenance of records and accounts of advancing nursing development and trends
Longitudinal studies of advanced nursing practice

Figure 6.8 Advanced Practice Nursing International Research Agenda. (Source: Key Informants, personal communication.)

agenda forward. Studies examining and providing a solid foundation of knowledge as to clinical outcomes will greatly enhance credibility in this field as key stakeholders evaluate the multiple changes and needs occurring in health systems worldwide.

Conclusion

At this stage in the evolution of research pertaining to advanced nursing practice, the question presents as to whether the data and results of current publications can be generalised beyond the reported study settings. There is interest in identifying a body of knowledge that drives advanced nursing practice. Key informants (personal communication) have made recommendations for an international research agenda that are diverse and insightful while emphasising the limitations of current knowledge. The comprehensiveness of the suggested global research agenda reflects the emergent nature of advanced nursing practice. Nurses at all levels are encouraged to become involved in some facet of the research process. The authors propose that an action-oriented and collaborative approach based on confidence in nursing and its associated principles is needed to accomplish a relevant research agenda for future development.

References

American Association of Colleges of Nursing. (1996). *The Essentials of Master's Education for Advanced Practice Nursing.* Washington, D.C.: Author.

American Nurses Association. (1996). *Scope and standards of advanced practice registered nursing.* Washington DC: Author.

Brehaut, J.D., Juzwishin, D. (2005). *Bridging the gap: The use of research in policy development.* Health Technology Assessment Unit, Initiative #18, Alberta Heritage Foundation for Medical Research: Author.

Brown, S.J. (2005). Direct clinical practice. In A.B. Hamric, J.A. Spross, C.M. Hanson (Eds) *Advanced practice nursing: An integrative approach*, 3rd Edition, pp. 143–185. St. Louis: Elsevier Saunders.

Buchan, J., Calman, L. (2004). *Skill-mix and policy change in the health workforce: Nurses in advanced roles*, OECD Health Working Papers No. 17, DELSA/ELSA/WD/HEA, 8.

Buchan, J., Dal Poz, M.R. (2002). Skill mix in the health care workforce: Reviewing the evidence. *Bulletin of World Health Organization*, 80(7), 575–580, Geneva: WHO.

Camiah, S. (1997). Utilization of nursing research in practice and application strategies to raise research awareness amongst nurse practitioners: a model for success. *Journal of Advanced Nursing*, 26, 1193–1202.

Champion, V.L., Leach, A. (1989). Variables related to research utilization in nursing. *Journal of Advanced Nursing*, 14, 705–710.

Closs, S.J., Cheater, F.M. (1994). Utilization of nursing research: culture, interest and support. *Journal of Advanced Nursing*, 19(4), 762–773.

De Back, V. (2005). *Writing for journals: the INR manual for nurse authors.* Geneva: International Council of Nurses.

De Palma, J.A., McGuire, D.B. (2005). Research. In A.B. Hamric, J.A. Spross, C.M. Hanson (Eds), *Advanced practice nursing: an integrative approach*, 3rd Edition, pp. 257–300. St. Louis: Elsevier Saunders.

Fawcett, J., Newman, D.M., Mcallister, M. (2004). Advanced practice nursing and conceptual models of nursing. *Nursing Science Quarterly*, April **17**(2), 135–138.

Fawcett, J., Watson, J., Neuman, B., Hinton Walker, P., Fitzpatrick, J.J. (2001). On nursing theories and evidence. *Journal of Nursing Scholarship*, **33**(2), 115–119.

Gardner, G., Carryer, J., Dunn, S., Gardner, A. (2004). *Nurse practitioner standards project: Report to Australian Nursing Council*. Australian Nursing Council: Author.

Hagedorn, S., Quinn, A.A. (2004). Theory-based NP practice: caring in action. *Topics in Advanced Practice Nursing ejournal*, **4**(4), Medscape.

Hickey, J.V. (2000). Advanced practice nursing at the dawn of the 21st century: Practice, education and research. In J.V. Hickey, R.M. Ouimette, S.L. Venegoni (Eds), 2nd Edition, *Advanced practice nursing: Changing roles and clinical applications*, pp. 3–33. Philadelphia: Lippincott Williams & Wilkins.

Holzemer, W. (1998). (Ed) *Practical guide for nursing research*. Geneva: International Council of Nurses: Author.

Hughes, F., Clarke, S., Sampson, D.A., Fairman, J., Sullivan-Marx, E.M. (2003). Research in support of nurse practitioners. In M. Mezey, D.O. McGivern, E.M. Sullivan-Marx (Eds), *Nurse practitioners: Evolution of advanced practice*, 4th Edition, pp. 84–107. New York: Springer.

International Council of Nurses. (2005a). *International classification for nursing practice (ICNP®)*. Geneva: Author.

International Council of Nurses. *Nursing research. A tool for action*. Retrieved October 28, 2005 from http://www.icn.ch/resnet.htm

Kraus, V.L. (2000). The research basis for practice: the foundation of evidence-based practice. In J.V. Hickey, R.M. Ouimette, S.L. Venegoni (Eds) *Advanced practice nursing: changing roles and clinical applications*, 2nd Edition, pp. 317–329. Philadelphia: Lippincott Williams & Wilkins.

May, A.L., Mulhall, A., Alexander, C. (1998). Bridging the research–practice gap: exploring the research cultures of practitioners and managers. *Journal of Advanced Nursing*, **28**(2), 428–436.

McGee, P., Castledine, G. (2003). Future directions in advanced nursing practice in the UK. In P. McGee, G. Castledine (Eds) *Advanced nursing practice*, 2nd Edition, pp. 225–237. Oxford: Blackwell Publishing.

Nicoteri, J.O., Andrews, C. (2003). The discovery of unique nurse practitioner theory in the literature: Seeking evidence using an integrative review approach. *Journal of the American Academy of Nurse Practitioners*, **5**(11), 494–500.

Sharma, R.R. (Undated). *An Introduction to advocacy. Training guide*. Washington: SARA Project–Advocacy Academy for Educational Development.

Stocking, B. (1995). Why research findings are not used by commissions – what can be done about it? *Journal of Public Health Medicine*, **17**(4), 380–382.

Woods, L. (2000). *The enigma of advanced nursing practice*. Salisbury, Wilts: Mark Allen.

Chapter 7
Future prospects and critical challenges for advanced nursing practice

Introduction

Advanced nursing practice is at a crossroads. Organisations such as the World Health Organization (WHO) and the International Council of Nurses (ICN) repeatedly stress that nursing is an essential part of the health service, and endorse the benefits of health care delivery provided by nurses and midwives. Chapter 1 indicates that governments, WHO and others now recognise that advanced nursing practice can make a significant contribution to the health of populations. It is now up to the profession to take up this challenge and develop pathways for advanced nursing practice commensurate to countries' health needs, and their aspirations for populations to enjoy the benefits of good health.

As in many new ventures, the future ahead rests on meeting a complex set of needs and dealing with environmental factors. The more urgent the demand for access to services, the more likely it is that advanced nursing practice will be considered as a part of the solution to improving the health of populations. Excess of physicians, confusion surrounding role implementation, lack of leadership, and financial and regulatory barriers contribute to a more slowly evolving process of acceptance.

The point of origin for the spark that starts the cascade of change may differ. It may be the inspired individual nurse with a vision of how nurse-managed services can improve care; or a physician or administrator who understands that collaborative models may make better use of the potential of the different health professionals when dealing with more complex health needs. An organisation or health care facility looking to enhance the cost-effectiveness of health services and improve quality can initiate changes to introduce skill-mixes that include the use of advanced practice nurses (APNs). A health care consumer exposed to advanced nursing in another facility or country can stimulate discussion on the need for a similar service in their community. A group of nurses searching for career pathways that enable them to expand their professional and clinical skills and be recognised for these efforts can be the catalyst for innovative progress which leads to the recognition and implementation of advanced practice roles (key informants, personal communication).

Future prospects

Preparing a health care workforce for the 21st century

Health care policy makers and planners are actively pursuing options for health care that are less reliant on the hospital sector but are at the same time creating a more responsive system of health care providers. They are looking at new ways of working and are searching for strategies that focus on the enhancement of primary care – the first point of contact with health care services. Training and educating professionals for different roles and a multidisciplinary approach appears to be emerging. (Department of Health, Social Services & Public Safety, Northern Ireland, 2005; Health and Medical Development Advisory Committee, Hong Kong, 2005; World Health Organization [WHO], (2005). Advanced practice nurses are in an ideal position to participate in the development of new health workforce strategies for the 21st century.

Primary health care services

Provision of adequate primary health care (PHC) services is being increasingly highlighted internationally. Central to this attention 'lie issues of political significance to policymakers, professional and workforce managers concerning who leads and who follows in the new emerging health service' (Williams, 2000, p. 3). There is growing evidence that more efficient and effective services can be delivered by closer cooperation among different professionals within PHC. The future prospect of working more closely together as nurses and other professionals take on the team approach and address PHC issues mandates that the individual professional roles will have to change and evolve, and education needs to shift its focus to prepare health care providers with the required knowledge and skills.

Opportunities for nurses to work differently will probably include entering not only primary health care settings but into specialties, new fields of practice and practice settings unfamiliar to nurses used to working mainly in hospitals. With attention directed to primary care and care provision in community settings examples of future developments and opportunities include:

- Primary health care in residential care homes for the elderly
- Family health care for all family members as a unit of care
- Expansion of community mental health and learning disabilities services
- Twenty-four hour crises response services and other telephone linked care
- Increased emphasis on health promotion, social well-being and disease prevention
- Multidisciplinary teams in specialised areas such as diabetes, respiratory illness, heart disease and cancer care
- Increased range of services provided at home
- The 'one-stop-shop' concept based on a wide range of services located in one centre e.g. physicians, APNs, pharmacists, physiotherapists, social workers and dieticians all together under one roof
- Advances in genomics, new gene therapies and antibiotics, and new effective therapies with an increased need for primary care providers (including APNs) in out-of-hospital centres (Department of Health, Social Services and Public Safety, 2005).

Chronic conditions and home care

The World Health Organization (2005) in attempting to meet the challenge of chronic conditions worldwide proposes the need for a new perspective that includes core competencies for all providers caring for patients with chronic conditions. The competencies include: patient-centred care, partnering, quality improvement, information and communication technology, and a public health perspective. Emphasis in this approach is placed on partnering in provision of care for chronic conditions in the hope that fragmented care could be decreased, thus improving care results. This transformation in the health care workforce will require additional education and training in an attempt to manage better the needs of populations who suffer from a chronic disease. Competent APNs will have an excellent opportunity to participate in an improved approach to chronic health care options.

Advanced practice nurses participating in the health care workforce for the 21st century would do well to heed the recommendation of WHO (2005) to 'emphasise management over cure, and long-term over episodic care' (p. 51). Core competencies to improve care for chronic conditions as identified by WHO are underpinned by the assumptions that:

- The essence of this care is to centre on the patient.
- Solo practice is no longer adequate to achieve positive outcomes for chronic problems.

- The workforce needs skills that ensure continuous quality improvement in terms of patient safety and service delivery efficiency.
- The ability to use available information and communication technology is essential.
- The workforce needs the ability to view health from a broad public health perspective (WHO, 2005, pp. 51–52).

Consistent with this emphasis is the return to, and the increased interest in some areas of the world in community development and home care in promoting continuity for health care. Again APNs are well placed to bear in mind this prospect when considering career choices for the future. Topics to consider will be what the position of APNs is in community health and home care, and what skills and knowledge are appropriate for working in these settings. Already in many parts of the world nurses are the main providers of PHC. As nurses and APNs work with communities their visibility and actions have the potential for contributing to 'healthy communities and sustainable development' (Nickson, 2004).

Technology and telehealth

Infrastructure for care is changing and the nurse looking to take up an APN role will be faced with a necessity to be literate in an ever widening range, and increasing sophistication of telecommunication technology and informatics. Access to the internet will affect how services are delivered and accessed. The public increasingly uses internet services as a source of information, but in the future technology will be used more often as an interactive way to communicate between individuals and their health care team in the self-management of chronic conditions, infections or communicable disease control. Telenursing will be an essential way for nurses to manage and provide health care services (Milholland, 2000).

Milholland (2000) points out that although technology and telehealth options can be seen as a method to facilitate public access to health care providers, increased use of technologies carry with them intended and unintended consequences, for example increased liability, challenges in communication and the requirement to refine and update skills and practice. APNs who are strategically placed to actively participate in distance technologies will need to be alert to legal and regulatory implications as well as standards and competencies for services delivered in this manner. The International Council of Nurses (Milholland, 2001) has provided comment on implications for nurses using telecommunications stating that there is an expectation that integration of technological options will ensure safety and quality of telenursing practice. While the American Nurses Association (1999) and specialty organisations in the United States provide recommended competencies for the nurse using telecommunication technologies, a recommendation is made that the competencies must be reviewed and adapted for specific settings. APNs in the future will be increasingly called upon to integrate their advanced knowledge and clinical skills with the heightened presence of useful and usable health care technologies.

Nurse entrepreneurs

The greater level of confidence and higher degree of autonomy being experienced by some APNs appears to be crystallising into a desire for increased independence and a subsequent affinity the entrepreneurial model (key informants, personal communication). Thus, as APNs gain confidence in the value of, and ability to deliver, nurse-based care as well as offering a widening range of services, a small but growing number will look to independent practice. In the ICN guidelines for the nurse entrepreneur, Saunders and Kingma (2004) describe nurse entrepreneurship as the involvement of nurses who own or sell products or services which may include:

- Nursing services e.g. independent clinical practice, nurse-owned facilities such as homes for the elderly
- Legal services e.g. reviewers or witness services in litigation
- Agencies and individuals providing specialised consultation on health care and health policy strategies
- Health care and health policy publications.

APNs venturing into entrepreneurial activities will need to learn and undertake a number of additional roles linked to business, risk management, and legislative and regulatory aspects of practice in addition to the services they provide. The recognition of the value of nurses functioning in this capacity is growing, acknowledging that nurse entrepreneurship has the potential of becoming a reliable and effective option in the diversity of approaches to health care delivery and related activities. Nurse entrepreneurs providing direct patient services should enter this pursuit 'with the understanding that entrepreneurship must adapt to the legislative, financial and political realities and expectations of the country, province or locality' (Saunders & Kingma, 2004, p. 6). For instance it means that health systems and clients recognise that the services provided by the nurse are directly reimbursable. APNs of the future will probably have increasing opportunities to explore possibilities of greater independence in practice, but they must be present to 'frame the issues and shape the debate to benefit quality patient care, and nursing independence' (Saunders & Kingma, 2004, p. 57).

Critical challenges

Throughout this book we have seen that at an international level advanced nursing practice is struggling to emerge, often venturing into territory that is uncharted and hostile. We have also seen that regardless of the hurdles, APNs are succeeding in many ways and under very different circumstances to make their presence felt. As ICN has shown through its programmes and projects, we have the tools to reach across time and geographical boundaries to learn from and assist each other, to share experiences, and to agree on common values and core standards for nursing. However, for APNs to fulfil their potential the authors believe that four critical challenges lie ahead: integrating APNs into the workforce, consensus building, capacity building and finding the evidence for the benefits of APN services.

Critical challenge 1: integrating advanced practice nurses into workforce planning

In the preceding chapters, it has been argued that to establish and sustain the distinctive services provided by advanced practice nurses (APNs), there needs to be a regulatory/legislative framework, an established scope of practice, and agreed standards for education and practice. These are insufficient in themselves without more deliberate planning for and development of human resources for health. The authors believe that if the APN is to become a permanent part of the nursing workforce, it is crucial that health human resources planning and development takes account of the place of advanced practice nursing in the health care spectrum. The APN needs to be an option when staff and skills-mix decisions are under consideration.

Affara and Styles (1992) point out that the aim of nursing resource planning is 'to ensure the presence of the right nurse with the right qualification at the right role at the right time, in the right place with the proper authority and appropriate recognition' (p. 80). Nursing resource planning needs to be placed within the broader system in which health care services operate, for it is the social, economic and political contexts that determine the requirements for health care services (O'Brien-Pallas *et al.*, 2005). National health policies and priorities, the state of development of the nursing profession, available resources (financial and human), APN education requirements, and a willingness to establish positions are important when deciding how to integrate advanced nursing practice within a health system. To begin to bring some order to the way APNs are prepared and introduced, nurses have to provide credible data on this category of health care provider to inform policy and planning decisions on roles, functions, pattern of utilisation, numbers and career pathways. Figure 7.1 demonstrates the relationship among the different players in the health system. While aspects such as scope of practice and standards are a major responsibility of the regulatory body, they cannot be developed without inputs from those responsible for overall human resources planning, development and management (HRPD & M), and more specifically those dealing with nursing resources. Questions such as the health context, health goals and priorities, unmet needs and fiscal issues will all be areas that are taken account of during the process of HRPD & M. The outcome of decisions will impact on roles and functions assigned to APNs, numbers required, where they will be practising, what authority is given, and the type of education and regulatory framework required.

Nursing workforce planning is currently high on the agenda of ministries of health. In the United Kingdom the National Health Service spends around two billion pounds sterling on training and education of clinical staff, but has recognised '. . . that current workforce planning and development arrangements

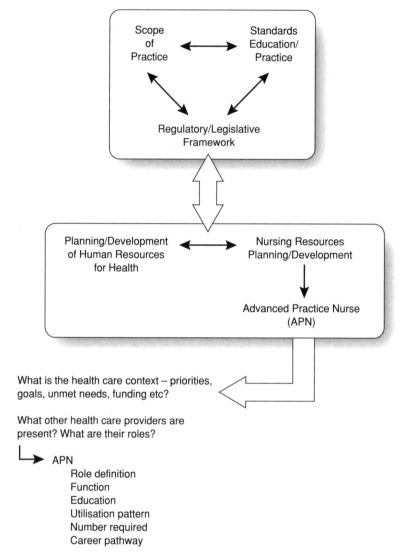

Figure 7.1   Relationship of evolution of advanced practice nurses to human resources planning and development. (Adapted from Affara & Styles, 1992, p. 74.)

inhibit the development of multi-professional planning and have not supported the creative use of staff skills' (Department of Health, 2000, p. 6). As O'Brien *et al.* (2005) point out, what is needed are 'strategies based on sound theoretical frameworks and methodologies . . . to effectively plan for and manage the nursing workforce and other health care providers' (p. 30).

The critical challenge for advanced nursing practice is to begin to understand and contribute to development of theoretical frameworks and methodologies that take account of the potential services that advanced nursing can bring to health care systems. Providing information and developing workforce methodologies are important, but they alone cannot achieve results. Activism and advocacy are required on the part of APNs to promote their role in health systems in order to establish strategies and create sustained working partnerships with policy- and decision-makers for integrating APNs within the health workforce.

Critical challenge 2: international consensus-building around definitions, scope of practice, core competencies and education

Previous chapters in this book have highlighted the considerable degree of uncertainty, confusion and incoherence surrounding many aspects of advanced nursing practice. This ambiguity touches even basic characteristics such as role definition, standards for education and titles. A lack of clarity exists within countries and across geographical borders. Therefore, it is not surprising that, as the concept of advanced nursing practice spreads from countries where roles are well established to those countries with little or no experience of the role, inconsistencies and differences begin to be important. They count because they are incompatible to a systematic, consistent and appropriate development of the role internationally.

Differences and inconsistencies are handicaps in a world where globalisation is taking place within a context of increased international trade in services and greater mobility of health professionals. The application of new technologies and expanding telecommunications has opened up new opportunities such as telehealth, telenursing and e-education, as well as openings and opportunities to work in, and learn from, other countries. Chapters 4 and 5 of this book referred to the process used by the Australian and New Zealand nursing regulation authorities to arrive at consensus over definitions, scope and standards. This was driven by a bilateral trade agreement. In the European Union the political decision to increase the movement of goods, services and persons among countries obliges nursing to arrive at a certain level of consensus on definitions and standards for the profession (Affara, 2004).

Networking is a way to achieve international consensus building. It enables communication to occur beyond organisational and national boundaries. The main goal of the ICN International Nurse Practitioner/Advanced Practice Nursing Network (INP/APNN) is 'to become an international resource for nurses practising in nursing practitioner (NP) or advanced practice nursing (APN) roles, and interested others (e.g. policymakers, educators, regulators, health planners)' (ICN, 2005). As the network evolves it is becoming clear that its role as a consensus-building forum should be one of its foremost priorities. This speaks directly to the determination of APNs to have a national and global identity. Therefore, the network goals (Figure 7.2) are important in assisting with adapting and applying the commonly held standards across geographic and health system boundaries.

The network has made progress by facilitating consensus on a definition of the APN, as described in Chapter 1, and role characteristics as delineated in

- Identify issues early and monitor how they develop.
- Follow trends.
- Offer special expertise through creating a resource pool from network members.
- Disseminate ICNs' and others' work in the field.
- Organise meetings and conferences.

Figure 7.2   ICN International Nurse Practitioner/Advanced Practice Nursing Network (INP/APNN) Goals.

Chapter 2. At the time of writing the network is in the process of identifying an international APN scope of practice, standards and core competencies.

The critical challenge is to find effective and durable mechanisms that allow for the continual building and updating of international agreement around core areas pertaining to the advanced practice role. In doing so advanced practice nursing needs to acknowledge the diversity of APN practice around the world, and find ways of recognising the multiple contributions of international nursing. This critical challenge speaks directly to the aspiration that APNs have a national and global identity that allows populations to identify who APNs are, and society to know and trust the services they offer.

Critical challenge 3: capacity building to strengthen advanced nursing practice in health systems internationally

Many key informants (personal communication) commented that, while there is a desire to advance more quickly in educating for and implementing advanced nursing practice roles, progress is slow and halting. Many of the barriers to progress have been discussed in previous chapters, but it is notable how many are due to an inability of individuals or organisations to perform those functions and tasks that would move them towards their strategic goals. In advanced nursing practice this is illustrated in a poor understanding of the role by leaders within and outside nursing; difficulties in making policy and structural changes to remove regulatory, policy and organisational impediments in order to integrate APNs into the health workforce; and timidity in introducing new competencies and practice models better suited to 21st century health challenges. Education is hampered by lack of understanding of the implication of changes in health care needs for programmes preparing nurses, a scarcity of suitable faculty, an absence of clinical role models, and a profession that clings to traditional models of professional education. The authors believe that all these relate in some way to deficits or a lack of capacity in individuals, organisations or systems to produce appropriate, effective and sustainable strategies, actions and consequently outcomes with respect to educating, regulating and using APNs.

Capacity building is poorly understood and tends to be equated only with the training of individuals. Milèn (2001) points out that thinking about capacity building or development has moved from the training focus to a 'continuing process of strengthening of abilities to perform core functions, solve problems, define and achieve objectives, and understand and deal with development needs' (p. 1). It could mean strengthening of links and development of the environments within which organisations exist through means such as bringing together organisations in one country to share information and provide a more effective lobbying voice, or embarking on a deliberate process of institutional building. Eventually capacity building should lead to independence as it increases the range of people, organisations and groups with knowledge, skill and confidence to identify problems and act on solutions.

One of the striking messages communicated by key informants (personal communication) is the dearth of experienced, knowledgeable nurses capable of acting strategically and effectively in policy and regulatory development; education; in creating good models for APN practice; and setting up advanced practice services adapted to be consistent with the needs and imperatives of health systems. Thus nursing fails to plan, act and find sufficient resources to tackle problematic areas such as:

- Gaining acceptance from nursing, other health professionals, health authorities and the public
- Overcoming legislative and regulatory barriers and acquiring a strong legal basis for APN practice
- Providing education pertinent to the scope of knowledge, characteristics and level of responsibilities expected of APNs
- Negotiating suitable clinical career pathways and positions that use APN capabilities to the full extent of preparation
- Securing commensurate salaries, fees, reimbursement and indemnity insurance.

The theme running through key informants (personal communication) comments was that paying attention to culture, values and power relations that influence organisations and individuals, and complementing and building on, not replacing, the strengths and capacities that already exist must underlie all capacity building efforts.

Various approaches are used in capacity building, ranging from the conventional methods of training and education and use of external national or international technical experts or consultants, to different forms of cooperation. Decades of experience by international organisations point to better results when approaches that build on collaboration through partnership are used, where partners work together to clarify and define the means to achieve goals. More recently interest has focused on the use of a variety of twinning arrangements to create partnership and collaboration (UNDP, 1997; Milèn, 2001). One of the lessons learned is that in capacity building interventions, poor ownership by the local partner is an important reason for unsustainable outcomes.

This critical challenge asks the nursing profession to be innovative and practical in engaging in activities of mutual assistance that increase the capacity of systems and the profession to sustain advanced nursing practice. Models for partnership, twinning and networking; sharing innovative and demonstrated methodologies; identifying the type of capacity development for individuals and institutions that result in sustainable educational programmes, regulatory frameworks and practice models; and finding the resources to carry out this work are significant aspects of the challenge.

Critical challenge 4: defining the gaps and finding the evidence

A key challenge facing advanced nursing practice is to come up with research capable of making available relevant and usable findings. The benefits that advanced nursing practice brings to health care systems and the health care workforce will be strengthened considerably by the presence of sound research data and publication of study findings. Key respondents (personal communication) over and over again request data that demonstrate the influence APNs have in provision of health care services. Increasingly the culture of health care is demanding evidence as the basis for decision and policy making. It is no longer good enough to offer opinions, examples of past practice and precedence (Kraus, 2000). Data from both a quantitative and qualitative research perspective are required to initiate comprehensive strategies based on sound frameworks presenting effective techniques that advocate for the presence of advanced nursing roles within varied health care settings.

Key stakeholders are asking questions such as: Why do nurses need to be educated at university level? Will nurses be lost to clinical practice in the wards with this level of education? Will introduction of APNs make the health care system more expensive? What do APNs add to quality health care provision? (key informants, personal communication). Convincing answers to common and practical questions must be supplied. Definitive answers that make sense within the context from which they arise are needed.

Chapter 6 in this book deals with why nurses require research competencies and need to be increasingly involved in research activities. Suggestions are given on a variety of ways for APNs to be regularly associated with inquiry and studies supportive of the conduct of research and practice utilisation. Listed throughout this book and in the research agenda, the areas requiring rigorous research are extensive and diverse.

Three important aspects of this critical challenge are:

- The support of research as being an integral part of advanced nursing practice workforce planning, practice development and policy formulation
- The creation of research alliances and the undertaking of collaborative research across institutions and health care systems
- The availability of research funding.

The authors strongly advocate for an international environment in which researchers from a variety of backgrounds can exchange ideas and collaborate on research in order to provide evidence on advanced nursing practice to health professionals, policy makers and consumers. The drive toward evidence-based practice, the changing roles of nurses and the implementation of clinical and research governance frameworks in many countries provides some indication of the vigorous and critical nature of this challenge (Freshwater, 2003). One goal advocated by the authors is the promotion of critical thinking and informed debate around the contextual and professional issues impacting and influencing advanced nursing practice. To fuel discussion and debate, improved access to balanced, diverse information based on research findings is essential in promoting enlightened decision-making that truly represents the important issues surrounding advanced nursing practice.

Conclusion

This chapter has described the potential for advanced nursing practice to thrive in some of the areas that are emerging as being important to health systems around the world in the 21st century. Multiple factors influence the consideration of integrating APNs into the health care environment. An international consensus on the determining factors essential for these nursing roles has the potential for becoming a driving force for discussion, debate and role clarification. Capacity building within systems worldwide can promote the idea that advanced nursing practice is realistic and do-able for numerous nurses and health care environments. Research that takes into consideration the research agenda presented in Chapter 6 will provide a stronger foundation of evidence to highlight this exciting advancement of nursing services worldwide.

The enthusiasm and energy generated by the prospect of expanding nursing services and the prospects for APNs to carve out a place in the health care systems of the future are many. However, does this phenomenon represent an identity crisis for nursing with a risk that pursuing it further will lead to professional confusion, or is it a sign of nursing progressing and responding to current and future health care demands?

The authors propose that the opportunities opening up due to health care reform, and efforts to re-orient efforts to the infinitely more complex and long-term constellation of health problems facing health care providers, do open up opportunities for nursing to pursue a proactive, targeted and sustainable development of advanced nursing practice. However, establishing a critical mass of APNs, with a clear identity and a capacity to demonstrate effectiveness and confidence in roles and responsibilities that are identified with APN practice implies that certain conditions exist. It means that advanced nursing practice is able to embrace the diversity of health care systems worldwide without losing its core characteristics. It entails the presence of international consensus on scope of practice founded on the core values of nursing, a scope that engages APNs in a range of advocacy, disease prevention, treatment and health promotion activities. It requires that advanced nursing practice demonstrates consistency across clinical and educational models adding new competencies that reflect dynamic changes in health care. It asks that APNs provide evidence that they are sustainable and valued health care providers, willing and able to provide that care in partnership with patients, their families, other health care providers and communities. It demands leadership, strategic thinking and concerted action to propel APNs into becoming acknowledged, necessary members of the health care team.

References

Affara, F.A. (2004). *Understanding mutual recognition agreements.* Geneva: International Council of Nurses.

Affara, F.A., Styles, M.M. (1992). *A nursing regulation guidebook: From principle to power.* Geneva: International Council of Nurses.

American Nurses Association. (1999). *Competencies for telehealth technologies in nursing.* Washington, D.C.: Author.

Department of Health. (2000). *A health service of all the talents: Developing the NHS workforce.* Consultation document on the review of workforce planning. London: Author. Retrieved 17 October, 2005 from http://www.dh.gov.uk/assetRoot/04/08/02/58/04080258.pdf

Department of Health, Social Services and Public Safety. (2005). *Primary health and social care: A strategic framework for the development of primary health and social care for individuals, families and communities in Northern Ireland.* Ref: 308/2004. Belfast: Author, Retrieved October 27, 2005 from http://www.dhsspsni.gov.uk

Freshwater, D. (2003). *Understanding and implementing clinical nursing research.* Paper distributed at the 2003 ICN biennial conference. Oxford: Blackwell Publishing.

Health and Medical Development Advisory Committee. (2005). *Building a healthy tomorrow. Discussion paper on the future of our health care system.* Health, Welfare and Food Bureau, Hong Kong Special Administrative Region Government. Full report available from http://www.hwfb.gov.hk/hmdac/

International Council of Nurses. (2005). *International Nurse Practitioner/Advanced Practice Nursing Network (INP/APNN). Aims and objectives.* Retrieved 21 October, 2005 from http://icn-apnetwork.org/

Kraus, V. (2000). The research basis for practice: The foundation for evidence-based practice. In J.V. Hickey, R.M. Ouimette, S.L. Venegoni (Eds) *Advanced practice nursing: changing roles and applications*, 2nd edition, pp. 317–329. Baltimore: Lippincott Williams & Wilkins.

Milèn, A. (2001). *What do we know about capacity building? An overview of existing knowledge and good practice.* Geneva: World Health Organization. Retrieved 20 October, 2005 from http://www.afronets.org/pubview.php/34/

Milholland, D.K. (2000). *Telehealth and telenursing: Nursing and technology advance together.* [Monograph # 4]. Geneva: International Council of Nurses.

Milholland, D.K. (2001). *International professional standards for telenursing programmes.* Geneva: International Council of Nurses.

Nickson, P. (2004). *Community development: Guidelines for action.* [Monograph 18], Geneva: International Council of Nurses.

O'Brien-Pallas, L., Duffield, C., Tomblin Murphy, G., Birch, S., Meyer, R. (2005). Nursing workforce planning: mapping the policy trail. Issue 2. In *The Global Nursing Review Initiative* Geneva: International Council of Nurses.

Saunders, E.M., Kingma, M. (2004). *Guidelines on the nurse entre/intrapreneur providing nursing service.* [Monograph 11]. Geneva. International Council of Nurses.

United Nations Development Fund. (1997). *Capacity Development.* Technical Advisory paper No 2, Management Development and Governance Division, Bureau for Policy Development, New York, Author. Retrieved March 6, 2006 from http://magnet.undp.org/Docs/cap/Capdeven.pdf

Williams, A. (2000). *Nursing, medicine and primary care.* Buckingham: Open University Press.

World Health Organization. (2005). *Preparing a health care workforce for the 21st century: The challenge of chronic conditions.* Geneva: Author.

Appendix 1
Key informant survey on advanced nursing practice (ANP) self-administered questionnaire

[Please first SAVE this questionnaire on your computer/network before completing it to ensure the data you enter is not lost]

Please complete and return electronically if possible by _____ to:

To ensure we have the correct information, please complete the following:

Title (Prof; Dr; Mr; Mrs; Miss; Ms; Other):

Surname/Family Name:

First Name:

Institution:

Title/Position:

Full Mailing Address:

Phone (include country and city code):

Fax (include country and city code):

e-mail:

Please describe the context to which your responses refer (e.g. country and/or region, field or focus of ANP)

What is your present relationship to ANP?

Definition

For the purposes of this questionnaire we are using the ICN definition. An advanced practice nurse is a registered nurse who has acquired the expert knowledge base, complex decision-making skills and clinical competencies for expanded practice, the characteristics of which are shaped by the context and/or country in which s/he is credentialed to practice. A Masters degree is recommended for entry level.

PART 1   HISTORY

Please give us a brief history of the introduction and evolution of advanced nursing practice in your context. Below are some of the areas you may wish to address amongst others.

- When was APN practice introduced?
- What were the factors leading to the development of APN role/s?
- Where was the role first introduced, and who was involved in initiating (e.g. was it practice, education or policy driven and supporting APN roles?)
- What were the challenges and how were they dealt with?

PART 2   THE ROLE

2.1   Is there an official definition of *advanced practice nursing* **and** *advanced practice nurse*?

Yes   ❑   No   ❑

If yes, we would appreciate if you would provide the definitions

Advanced Practice Nursing

Advanced Practice Nurse

2.2   Below are a number of characteristics included in ICN's definition of the APN. Please check those applying to your situation.

- ❑   Integrates research, education, practice and management
- ❑   High degree of professional autonomy and independent practice
- ❑   Case Management/own caseload
- ❑   Advanced health assessment skills, decision-making skills and diagnostic reasoning skills
- ❑   Recognised advanced clinical competencies
- ❑   Provision of consultant services to health providers
- ❑   Plans, implements & evaluates programs
- ❑   Recognised first point of contact for clients
- ❑   Other, please specify:

2.3   In what areas do APNs practice?

- ❑   Primary health care/Community health
- ❑   Home care
- ❑   Paediatrics
- ❑   Adult care
- ❑   Obstetric care

❑ Maternity care
❑ Mental health
❑ Anaesthesiology
❑ Critical care
❑ Elderly care
❑ Long term care
❑ Other, please specify

Let us know anything more about the role of the APN which is important to you in your situation.

PART 3 EDUCATION

If a formal education for APN exists can you let us know the following

3.1 What are the entry requirements?

3.2 How long (in MONTHS) is the APN programme?

_____ Months

3.3 What ACADEMIC qualification is earned on completion of the APN?

❑ Diploma
❑ Baccalaureate
❑ Masters
❑ Other, please specify

3.4 Are programmes preparing APNs accredited?

Yes ❑   No ❑

If yes, tell us by whom

3.5 Who participate in setting standards and competencies for APN?

❑ Government:
  Please specify:
❑ Regulatory authority/ies:
  Please specify:
❑ Nursing profession:
  Please specify:
❑ Others, please specify:

Let us know anything more about the education of the APN which is important to you in your situation.

PART 4   REGULATION

4.1   Is Advanced Nursing Practice regulated?

Yes   ❑   No   ❑

If **YES**

4.2   What kind of credential is awarded?

❑   Registration
❑   Certification
❑   Licensure
❑   Other, please specify:

4.3   Is the regulatory/credentialing body, which registers and/or licenses generalist nurses for practice:

❑   National government or a governmental agency?
❑   Sub-national/regional government or agency (state/province/canton etc.)?
❑   Local government or agency?
❑   Not part of a government body?

4.4   If it is non-governmental, what kind of an organisation is it?

❑   Linked to one (or more) professional nursing organisation/s **with** delegated legal authority to regulate
❑   Linked to one (or more) professional nursing organisation/s **without** delegated legal authority to regulate
❑   Other, please specify:

4.5   What title is the regulated APN authorised to use?

4.6   If advanced practice nursing is NOT regulated, please list the titles that are used by nurses who are practising in this role?

4.7   What processes are used to validate attainment of required standards/competencies/other requirements for registration/licensure? (You may select more than one)

❑   Acquiring educational diploma/certificate/degree
❑   Clinical assessment
❑   Test/exams
❑   Practice requirements
❑   Self assessment
❑   Peer review
❑   Portfolio review
❑   Interview

❑ Review of transcripts
❑ References
❑ Other, please specify:

4.8 Is the credential (i.e. registration/licensure)

❑ Awarded for an indefinite period?
❑ Renewed periodically?
If renewed, how often? Every _____ Years

4.9 Which of the following exist in your country with respect to advanced nursing practice?

❑ Right to diagnose
❑ Authority to prescribe medication
❑ Authority to prescribe treatment
❑ Authority to refer clients to other professionals
❑ Authority to admit patients to hospital

4.10 What are the renewal requirements?

❑ Payment of a fee
❑ Meeting practice requirements
❑ Evidence of continuing education or professional development
❑ Other, please specify: ____

4.11 If practice requirements are necessary for renewal, what amount and type are specified?

Amount _____ Days (If stated in hours, translate into days using your country's calculation of number of hours equalling 1 day)

Type, if specified:

4.12 What evidence of continuing education or professional development is required, if any?

Amount _____ Days (If stated in hours, translate into days using your country's calculation of number of hours equalling 1 day)

Type, if specified:

PART 5 RESEARCH

5.1 Please let us know of any research (published or unpublished) you know of that is related to advanced practice nurses (practice, regulation education policy). We are particularly interested in research undertaken in your country. Please give us the title and full reference and how we may access this research.

5.2   If you were to develop a research agenda for advanced practice nursing, what would you include? Please indicate what you consider priority areas.

PART 6   OTHER ISSUES

6.1   What would you consider are the major challenges facing the development of advanced nursing practice in your country/region?

6.2   We are interested in strategies you have used or are continuing to use to introduce and develop advanced nursing practice. We would like to know of those that have proved successful and those that have failed, and what you think contributed to success or otherwise.

6.3   What do you think are the three most important actions that should be taken by the international nursing profession to promote and support advanced practice nursing?

We would appreciate it if you can share any concrete experiences met by advanced practice nurses during the initiation and development of the role and the introduction in the health care system and to the public.

For example: How you dealt with challenges – from other health care workers, policy makers, regulators
The impact of introducing APN on practice, client outcome

Please let us know of other persons you think will be useful key informants.

Please return the completed questionnaire by _____

Thank you for responding to this survey. We value your input into our thinking about this book, and helping us to take an international perspective.

Appendix 2
Scope of practice examples

Critical to advanced nursing practice development is defining the scope of practice. Scopes of practice provided here are examples used in nursing practice Acts in various countries or recommended by professional organisations.

Australia

Australian Capitol Territory (ACT)

Registration as a nurse practitioner in the ACT is in accordance with sections 12 and 13 of the Nurses Act 1988.

A nurse practitioner is a registered nurse working within a multidisciplinary team whose role includes autonomous assessment and management of clients using nursing knowledge and skills gained through advanced education and clinical experience in a specific area of nursing practise. The role may include but is not limited to the direct referral of the patients to other health care professionals, the prescribing of a designated and agreed list of medications, and the ordering of a designated and agreed list of diagnostic investigations (Nurses Board of the ACT. Retrieved 20 October, 2005 from http://www.nursesboard.act.gov.au/policy_practitioner.htm)

New Zealand

Nurse Practitioners are expert nurses who work within a specific area of practice incorporating advanced knowledge and skills. They practise both independently and in collaboration with other health care professionals to promote health, prevent disease and to diagnose, assess and manage people's health needs. They provide a wide range of assessment and treatment interventions, including differential diagnoses, ordering, conducting and interpreting diagnostic and laboratory tests and administering therapies for the management of potential or actual health needs. They work in partnership with individuals, families, whanau and communities across a range of settings. Nurse Practitioners may choose to prescribe medicines within their specific area of practice. Nurse Practitioners also demonstrate leadership as consultants, educators, managers and researchers and actively participate in professional activities, and in local and national policy development. The Nursing Council competencies for Nurse Practitioners describe the skills, knowledge and activities of Nurse Practitioners.

New Zealand Gazette, *15 September, 2004, No. 120 2959*

Dual country recommended scope of practice for Australia and New Zealand

The NP Standards Research Project recommended a scope of practice for Mutual Recognition Agreement purposes (New Zealand and Australia). It states that:

A nurse practitioner is a registered nurse educated to function autonomously and collaboratively in an advanced and extended clinical role. The NP role includes assessment and management of the clients using nursing knowledge and skills and may include but is not limited to the direct referral of patients to other health professionals, prescribing medications and ordering diagnostic investigations. The nurse practitioner role is grounded in the nursing profession's values, knowledge, theories and practice and provides innovative and flexible health care delivery that complements other health care providers. The scope of practice of the nurse practitioner is determined by the context in which the nurse practitioner is authorized to practise (p. 3).

Gardner, G., Carryer, J., Dunn, S., Gardner, A. (2004) Nurse Practitioner Standards Project. *Report to the Australian Nursing Council.*

Canada

There is no one definition or scope of practice for advanced nursing practice across Canadian provinces and territories. Scopes of practice provided are examples in legislative instruments from select provinces.

Northwest Territories and Nunavut

Nursing Profession Act, S.N.W.T. 2003, c.15, and amendments to the Nunavut Nursing Profession Act, came into force January 1, 2004:

In addition to the scope of practice of all RNs, a nurse practitioner using advanced knowledge, skills, and judgment may:

- *Make a diagnosis identifying a disease, disorder or condition*
- *Communicate a diagnosis to a patient*
- *Order and interpret screening and diagnostic tests authorised in guidelines approved by the Minister*
- *Select, recommend, supply, prescribe, monitor the effectiveness of drugs as authorized in guidelines approved by the Minister*

- *Perform other procedures that are authorized in guidelines approved by the Minister (p. 10).*

> *Retrieved 20 October, 2005 from*
> *http://www.justice.gov.nt.ca/PDF/ACTS/Nursing_Profession.pdf*

Ontario

> *An RN(EC) has advanced knowledge and decision-making skills in health assessment, diagnosis, therapeutics (including pharmacological, complementary and counselling interventions), health care management and community development and planning. Their scope of practice includes:*

- *assessing and providing services to clients of all developmental stages, and to families and communities; and*
- *providing comprehensive health services encompassing:*
  - *treatment of episodic illness and injuries;*
  - *identification and management of chronic stable conditions;*
  - *prevention of disease and injuries;*
  - *health promotion and education;*
  - *rehabilitation;*
  - *continuity of care; and*
  - *support services*

> *Source: College of Nursing of Ontario. (2005). Retrieved 28 June, 2006 from http://www.cno.org/docs/reg/4 5025_fsExtendedclass.pdf*

United States

As in Canada there is no one consistent scope of practice across the country. However the National Council of State Board defines a scope in its Model Practice Act.

> *The scope of an advanced practice registered nurse includes but is not limited to performing acts of advanced assessment, diagnosing, prescribing, selecting, administering and dispensing therapeutic measures, including over-the-counter drugs, legend drugs and controlled substances, within the advanced practice registered nurse's role and specialty appropriate education and certification.*

> *Source: National Council of State Boards. (2004). Model Nurse Practice Act. Retrieved from http://www.ncsbn.org/pdfs/chapter2.pd*

Scope recommended by a professional organisation

> *Nurse practitioners are primary care providers who practice in ambulatory, acute and long term care settings. According to their practice specialty these providers provide nursing and medical services to individuals, families and*

groups. In addition to diagnosing and managing acute episodic and chronic illnesses, nurse practitioners emphasize health promotion and disease prevention. Services include, but are not limited to ordering, conducting, supervising, and interpreting diagnostic and laboratory tests, and prescription of pharmacologic agents and non pharmacologic therapies. Teaching and counseling individuals, families and groups are a major part of nurse practitioner practice. Nurse practitioners practice autonomously and in collaboration with health care professionals and other individuals to diagnose, treat and manage the patient's health problems. They serve as health care researchers, interdisciplinary consultants and patient advocates.

Source: American Academy of Nurse Practitioners. (2002). Scope of practice for nurse practitioners. *Retrieved 20 October, 2005 from www.aanp.org*

Appendix 3
Strengths, Weaknesses, Opportunities, Threats (SWOT)

Strengths	Weaknesses
Evidence of competence of nurses working in advanced nursing practice roles, and managing complex health problems	Poor role definition
	Proliferation of titles
	Variable levels of role autonomy
Demonstrated acceptance by public	Significant variability in standards and quality of educational programmes for role preparation
Nursing commitment to develop clinical roles	Few mentors/role models in clinical setting
Demonstrated capability to provide most primary health care services and to act as entry point into the health system	Poorly prepared faculty
	Regulation lags behind practice
	Regulatory/legislative barriers
Nurses often the only available professional within reach	Inadequate understanding of advanced nursing practice by health policy makers, nurses, other health professional
Respected status for nursing	Poor acceptance as skilled practitioner by public
	Resistance to expanded role from physicians
Opportunities	**Threats**
Rising educational levels of nurses	Introduction of categories healthcare providers that may be seen to compete such as physician assistants
Move of nursing education to universities	Medical dominance
Emphasis on illness prevention and health promotion intervention	Absence of career pathways
Rising demand for management of chronic and long term illness	Lack of sufficient number of qualified faculty to prepare APNs
Governments' desire to improve health service coverage and reduce access barriers	Introduction of the role without clear definitions of scope of practice, and ensuring posts are designated for APNs
Shortage of physicians	Unavailability or insufficient funding for education, establishing posts and reimbursement of advanced practice nursing services
Re-assessment of scopes of practice as governments seek more efficient and effective use of health care workers	Difficulty in obtaining indemnity insurance
Interest in innovative health delivery models e.g. collaborative practice	

Sources: Key Informants

Appendix 4
Principles to guide standards development

(1) **Purpose:** Standards should be designed to achieve a stated purpose. The purpose needs to be explicit and relate to the target for the standards. Purpose may apply to the quality of services, educational programmes and products or the performance of health professionals.

(2) **Professional scope of practice and accountability:** Standards should be based upon clear definitions of professional scope of practice and accountability. As nurses and other health care professionals are accountable for the actions they take in the provision of care, standards should make responsibilities explicit and consistent with the legal, ethical and professional accountability of those to whom they apply.

(3) **Universal levels of performance:** Standards should promote universal levels of performance and encourage professional identity and mobility. Although variation between institutions and from country to country occur, and is desirable to adequately meet needs in a specific context, wide divergence in standards allows for development of inequalities in health care, stifles a broad and uniform development of the profession and reduces mobility of practitioners.

(4) **Flexibility:** Standards should be explicit enough to achieve their objective while allowing the flexibility to adapt to the local context, innovations, growth and change. Standards need to allow for flexibility to facilitate applicability at national or local levels or for their adaptation to changes in health care systems. There must be room to express standards according to local needs, without jeopardising the consistency of standards between the different levels.

(5) **Relevance:** Standards should address areas deemed important, and be applicable, and pertinent. Relevance of the processes used in all aspects of health care, including the education for practice, is necessary if there is to be effective and efficient attainment of goals.

(6) **Collaboration:** Standards should foster collaboration among professions offering essential services. Standards development must acknowledge the necessity for an integrated health care system that focuses on consumer driven services that meet people's needs. Growing emphasis on multidisciplinary health care delivery, partnerships and collaboration, and issues

of shared competencies and overlapping scope of practice are now emerging more strongly as increasingly health professionals work collaboratively and collegially, accepting shared responsibility and accountability for health care delivery.

(7)   **Cultural competence:** Standards should promote cultural competence. Building a nursing and health workforce and a health system that is sensitive to cultural needs is important if care obligations to all groups are to be met safely and competently. Standards are important tools in shaping systems and practice that respect and acknowledge the diversity of populations that health care systems serve.

(8)   **Consumer rights:** Standards should acknowledge realistic consumer expectations, and be developed with active participation of users of the services. Nurses and other health professionals acknowledge that any health delivery system should be consistent with realistic consumer expectations. Opportunities must be found for consumers' views to be seriously represented in standard setting. The model will vary from society to society as perceptions of who are considered legitimate consumer representatives, and the modalities for participation, may differ according to other cultural and societal traditions.

(9)   **Access and Equity:** Standards should promote greater equity and more access to health care. Standards may be used to exclude or contribute to improving access to service and equity in health care. One way to make standards more inclusive is to focus on consistency and comparability of issues that transcend differential resources.

(10) **Coherence and Consistency:** Standards should promote consistency; that is, standards that are uniform and compatible in different settings, places, and times, and consistent with the purpose of the specific related standards. Standards should clearly define their scope, i.e. the range of activities they cover. Consistency and comparability enhance the usefulness of standards allowing more meaningful comparison of an activity against another. They also promote clearer language and enhance the more uniform development of standards. The concepts of consistency and comparability are essential for the credibility of standards.

(11) **Convergence:** Standards promote efforts to reach consensus where differences in existing or developing standards in the same topic are reduced to a minimum or eliminated. The process of convergence involves the endeavour of reaching a consensus about a standard with a reduction of difference between current standards or developing standards. Convergence maximises the potential for international comparability in standards development.

(12) **Reliability:** Standards should represent what they claim to represent; that is, the fact, practice or action is correct or demonstrates what it

purports. Standards need to convey clearly intent to those implementing, measuring or evaluating standards. Such characteristics in standards increase the probability that similar conclusions will be reached about the standards. Vague, imprecise or cursory language inevitably produces confusion, and misunderstanding.

(13) Evaluation: Standards should be evaluated by an established and formalised review and monitoring process. For standards to achieve their purpose there is a need to systematically monitor the effect of application of standards. This includes putting in place a mechanism for seeking feedback from stakeholders and interested parties. Through evaluation, standards are more likely to remain relevant and undergo change as the situation alters.

(14) Measurement: Standards should be amenable to measurement of performance. Measurement of compliance with standards takes many forms, however, methods to use to measure performance should take account of cultural factors, the availability of expertise and resources to carry out the measures and interpret the results.

Adapted from Affara, F.A. & Percival, E. (2004). *International principles and framework for standards development in nursing*. Geneva: International Council of Nurses.

Appendix 5
Samples of course descriptions in an advanced nursing practice curriculum

Course title: Pathophysiology for advanced practice nursing

Course description

This course will provide a comprehensive, scientific background for the assessment, evaluation and advanced nursing management of processes resulting in manifestations of disease. A brief review of normal physiology and anatomy will be included. Emphases will be on the pathophysiology of selected disorders and diseases as examples of alterations of body systems when normal physiology and anatomy are impaired.

Course Objectives

Upon completion of this course, the student will be able to:

- Analyse the relationship between normal physiology and specific system alterations produced by disease processes
- Describe the aetiology, developmental considerations, pathogenesis and clinical manifestations of specific disease processes
- Discuss the purpose, results, interpretation of procedures and laboratory tests used in the diagnosis and management of clients with specific organ system alterations
- Utilise multiple resources to support critical thinking and decision making in assessing alterations in normal physiology.

Credits

According to the rules of the educational institution.

Prerequisites

Preparation at the generalist nurse level.

Teaching/learning strategies

Lecture, seminar discussions, small group work, case studies, oral presentations by students.

Course expectations

The faculty will serve as lecturer, resource and facilitator for the students in meeting course objectives. Emphases will be placed on class discussion and presentation of case studies and additional topics related to the course objectives. Each student will hand in a final copy of two case studies.

Evaluation criteria

Class participation, case studies (oral and written), brief frequent quizzes.

Textbooks/resources

Coursework will be based on access to multiple resources including additional texts, periodicals and internet resources. A required text and journal articles along with a list of recommended reading will be provided at the beginning of the course.

Course title: Pharmacology for advanced practice nursing

Course description

This course will provide the basis for understanding the use of pharmacotherapeutic agents at an advanced level. This is not an introductory pharmacology course. Content will be at a level appropriate to facilitate critical thinking as related to therapeutic management for APN students. Content will be organised around body systems and the main categories of drugs that impact the specific system. Topics will include information on therapeutics, adverse effects, and indications for use and drug interactions. Students will be expected to integrate knowledge of categories of drugs as it relates by system to the development of case studies and related drug management.

Course objectives

Upon completion of this course the student will be able to:

- Discuss the pharmacokinetic and pharmacodynamic actions of specified drugs
- Describe major pharmacological differences and indications for specific pharmacotherapeutic agents within a given drug category
- Analyse, identify and provide rationale for appropriate drug treatment given a specific clinical situation
- Incorporate the use of pharmacotherapeutic agents as one component of comprehensive care, with appropriate education application of relevant research and a holistic view of client's health status.

Credits

According to the rules of the educational institution.

Prerequisites

Preparation as a generalist nurse.

Teaching/learning strategies

Lectures, seminar discussions, case studies, small group work and student presentations of drug management.

Course expectations

Faculty will serve as a lecturer, resource and facilitator for the students in meeting course objectives. Emphases will be placed on class discussion and integration of content with case study discussions in the pathophysiology course. A case analysis approach will be the principal method of active learning.

Evaluation criteria

Class participation; first test – basic principles of pharmacology; short quizzes; case studies; final examination.

Textbooks/resources

Coursework will be based on access to multiple resources including additional texts, periodicals and internet resources. A required text and journal articles along with a list of recommended reading will be provided at the beginning of the course.

Course title: Primary care problems of adults

Course description

This course is structured to enable students to gain the problem-solving and clinical strategies necessary for practice as APNs. Course content will focus on the methodologies used to diagnose and treat common health problems and concerns including the educational and counselling components of care.

Objectives

Upon completion of this course, the student will be able to:

- Explore the role of the advanced practice nurse in screening, diagnosing and treating clients with common adult health problems
- Incorporate health care services and preventive health care teaching as appropriate for the patient's problem, cultural/ethnic background, and abilities
- Describe the aetiology, pathophysiology and presenting signs and symptoms of each disorder
- Identify the common differential diagnoses associated with each health problem
- Identify the laboratory analyses and diagnostic imaging appropriate for evaluating the client
- Select appropriate treatment modalities and management for the diagnosed problem incorporating a holistic, culturally sensitive approach
- Counsel the patient regarding health conditions in the context of his/her family, home, work and community environments
- Develop appropriate plans for follow-up care based on the patient's identified physiological and psychosocial needs
- Utilise current research to plan and evaluate management strategies.

Credits

According to the rules of the educational institution.

Pre-requisites

Pathophysiology and pharmacology at advanced level.

Criteria

Required for all APN students. Open to others with permission of the subject lecturer.

Teaching/learning strategies

Lectures, case study analyses and class discussion on selected topics.

Assessment

Written assignments, mid-term examination, final examination.

Textbooks/resources

Coursework will be based on access to multiple resources including additional texts, periodicals and internet resources. A required text and journal articles along with a list of recommended reading will be provided at the beginning of the course.

Course title: Advanced clinical practice for advanced nurse practitioners

Course description

This course is designed to provide real-life clinical experience in order to directly prepare the APN student for advanced clinical practice upon completion of a APN programme.

Objectives

- Develop case management skills at an advanced level within a real life setting
- Support clinical decisions with scholarly evidence
- Include pharmacological and non-pharmacological approach in management planning
- Establish collaborative skills with other health professionals
- Incorporate the health teaching and health promotion.

Credits

According to the rules of the educational institution.

Duration

16 weeks (4 months).

Pre-requisites

Successful completion of advanced health assessment, pharmacology, pathophysiology and adult health courses or theory to clinical practice.

Exclusions

This subject is not available to students who do not hold professional qualifications in nursing.

Learning approach

Supervised clinical practicum.

Assessment

Teaching is provided by the faculty member who has a major role in supervising the theoretical aspect of the practicum and the preceptor who has a primary role in working with, and acting as a mentor to, the student in the clinical attachment. The faculty member will make the final decision on the assessment grade in consultation with the preceptor, and the student where appropriate. The grade should reflect the competence of the student in defining clear goals, stating achievable outcomes, and fulfilling the objectives in developing the advanced practice nurse role. Based on the learning needs of the student, the faculty and preceptor together with the student will:

- Set clear and achievable learning outcomes
- Define practice hours and timings within the clinical setting
- Develop clinical logs reflective of clinical experience
- Present brief case studies from clinical experiences
- Communicate with faculty to schedule clinical site visits
- Arrange supervised clinical practice in laboratory setting if needed
- Provide clinical and case discussions in seminar settings

Course title: Theoretical approach to nursing

Course description

The focus of this course is on evaluating the factors and issues influencing the development of theory in nursing. The content will include the process of theory development as well as critical analysis of selected nursing theories and related theories from other biopsychosocial disciplines. Students will critique theories and explore their utilisation in nursing. Linkages among theory, practice and research will be explored.

Course Objectives

Upon completion of this course, the student will be able to:

- Analyse terminology associated with theory development
- Describe factors and issues influencing development of nursing theory
- Critically analyse differences between and among theories, models and conceptual frameworks in nursing
- Analyse relationships among theory, research and practice in nursing
- Apply selected criteria in the evaluation of a nursing theoretical formulation
- Critique and compare nursing theories
- Explore the utilisation of nursing theory in advanced clinical practice.

Credits

Determined by the teaching institution.

Prerequisites

Graduate student majoring in nursing.

Teaching/learning strategies

The class will be conducted in a seminar format and will include preparatory reading assignments, discussion, debate and student presentations. The faculty will serve as facilitator in fulfillment of course objectives.

Course expectations

Students will come to class prepared to discuss and debate the concept of theory development and how it applies to nursing practice as well as the learning environment in general. Each student will compare and contrast two nursing theories, models or conceptual frameworks. Each student will define criteria for evaluating nursing theory. Each student will present an example of the theoretical basis for nursing practice.

Evaluation criteria

Seminar preparation and participation, comparative paper, student led seminar presentation.

Caution: A caveat in giving a course based on the theoretical approach to nursing is that most current nursing theory is based on a Western approach and values. Therefore, in countries where these values do not necessarily fit their perspective, this course may be given in order to assist the student understand existing literature linking theory, research and practice. It is hoped that in the future, as the body of knowledge supportive of a theoretical approach to nursing expands beyond the strong western influences, it will embrace approaches that grow out of other cultures, values and ways of thinking about the person, the family, society, health and illness.

Course title: Advanced theoretical concepts in clinical care

Course Description

This course will focus on development of a knowledge base for clinical decision-making in the assessment, diagnosis and management of health problems across the life span. Topics will include health promotion and maintenance, disease prevention, diagnosis and treatment of common acute and stable chronic illnesses in adults.

Course objectives

Upon completion of this course the student will be able to:

- Analyse clinical problems related to the health of adults based on knowledge of human development and pathophysiological processes

- Using selected case studies, develop advanced practice nursing interventions directed toward health promotion, disease prevention and management of common acute and stable chronic illness in adults
- Develop strategies for consultation and collaboration with patients, families, professionals and others in the planning and delivery of care
- Formulate a plan of care based on patient history, physical assessment and diagnostic data
- Advance the practice of nursing through the use of appropriate theory and research.

Credit

Determined by the institution.

Prerequisites

Pathophysiology and pharmacology at an advanced level.

Teaching strategies

Weekly topic and case focused seminars using practice-based learning (PBL) format. The faculty is the facilitator with a focus on active student participation. Students are evaluated on evidence of critical thinking and progress toward informed advanced practice nursing care of adults. Additional integration of physical assessment skills at an advanced level and clinical experience to enhance learning will be included.

Evaluation criteria

Class attendance/participation, clinical case presentations (written and oral presentations), take home assignments (less complex case studies, take home examination or other projects related to the weekly seminar topic with an aim to increase learning and critical thinking rather than memorisation).

Appendix 6
Preceptor guidelines, student and preceptor evaluation forms

Defining advanced practice nurse

The advanced practice nurse is a registered nurse who has acquired the expert knowledge base, complex decision-making skills and clinical competencies for expanded practice. Central to the role are certain characteristics descriptive of the nature of practice. This includes:

- Ability to integrate research, education, practice and management
- High degree of professional autonomy
- Case management
- Advanced health assessment, decision-making and diagnostic reasoning skills
- Advanced clinical competencies
- Consultant services to other health care providers
- Ability to plan, implement and evaluate programs

Expectations of preceptors

As a clinician as well as an instructor, the preceptor will serve as a professional role model facilitating the advanced practice nursing student to achieve his/her learning objectives within the clinical setting. As development of clinical excellence is implicit in the clinical objectives, preceptors must be experienced clinicians. In this clinical teaching approach, a *consistent one-on-one relationship between the experienced practitioner and student* is built up so that oversight and support is available as the student acquires clinical skills at an advanced level. The preceptor will be provided with a copy of the practicum course description and the clinical learning outcomes.

Preceptors will be expected to:

(1) Enhance skill performance in relation to technical as well as cognitive skills (e.g. advanced level critical thinking and decision-making)
(2) Promote confidence and comfort for the student in the areas of:
   (a) History taking
   (b) Examination appropriate to the case
   (c) Testing & evaluation appropriate to the case

    (d) Assessment & differential diagnosis based on presenting concern, history, examination & other diagnostic testing

    (e) Development of a management plan & interventions

    (f) Appropriate case follow-up

    (g) Encouragement of review of evidenced based research as applicable to clinical decision-making.

Supervision by the preceptor should progress from observation of the preceptor by the student to more independent, autonomous activities based on the skill base of the student, complexity of the case and observation of the preceptor as to how the student role might best develop in each individual situation. It is expected the relationship between the student and preceptor will be based on mutual consultation and collaboration with backup and support from the school of nursing faculty responsible for this course.

    Students are expected to keep a daily patient log. Additionally, they will be participating in discussion and review at weekly seminars. Periodic site visits will be scheduled by the faculty for this course. Students will be evaluated for competency in history taking and performing physical examinations prior to assignment to a clinical setting. At the completion of the clinical assignment the preceptor will provide an evaluation of the student to the faculty, and the student will provide an evaluation of their clinical experience.

Preceptor Evaluation (to be completed by the student)

Name of preceptor: _____

Clinical setting: _____

Name of evaluator _____

Instructions: Rate your clinical preceptor on each item below, giving the highest score for unusually effective performances. Place the number that most nearly expresses your view in the blank before each statement. Provide comments as desired as evidence of your choice.

Highest			Average			Lowest
6	5	4	3	2	1	0

Place **NA** in the blank if the question is not applicable to the situation.

_____ 1. Provided introduction to the clinic, staff and essential policies and procedures.

_____ 2. Selected patients that provided opportunities to meet learning objectives.

_____ 3. Provided assistance and support in new and unfamiliar situations.

_____ 4. Provided me with helpful and timely feedback.

_____ 5. Provided a supportive learning environment to learn comfortably.

_____ 6. Answered questions freely.

_____ 7. Expressed willingness to help me learn.

_____ 8. Served as an appropriate role model for advanced clinical practice.

_____ 9. Encouraged me to be aware of professional accountability.

_____ 10. Identified additional resources to enhance my learning.

Share your comments about the following. Use the other side of the paper for more comments.

Would you recommend this preceptor to future students of this programme? Explain why or why not.

What behaviors of this preceptor do you believe to be exemplary?

What specific suggestions would you make concerning this preceptor?

Student Evaluation (to be completed by the preceptor)

Name of student: _____

Clinical setting: _____

Name of preceptor: _____

Instructions: Rate your clinical practicum student on each item below, giving the highest score for unusually effective performances. Place the number that most nearly expresses your view in the blank before each statement. Provide comments as desired as evidence of your choice.

Highest			Average			Lowest
6	5	4	3	2	1	0

Place **NA** in the blank if the question is not applicable to the situation.

_____ 1. Capacity to synthesize physiological, sociological and psychological factors.

_____ 2. Competence to conduct a history & physical examination appropriate to cases.

_____ 3. Proficiency at distinguishing variations of normal from abnormal with exam and assessment.

_____ 4. Demonstration of advanced level proficiency in assessment and management.

_____ 5. Expression of critical thinking as related to differential diagnoses.

_____ 6. Ability to respond positively to critique & comments from preceptor.

_____ 7. Demonstration of consultative and collaborative skills.

_____ 8. Knowledge of pharmacological as well as non-pharmacological strategies.

_____ 9. Awareness of professional accountability.

_____ 10. Ability to identify additional resources to enhance learning.

Provide your comments about the following. Use the other side of the paper for additional comments:

What behaviours of this student do you believe to be outstanding?

What specific suggestions would you make concerning this student?

Appendix 7
Checklist for authors preparing to submit an article for publication

Submission of an article implies that the work has not been published and is not being considered for publication elsewhere. Review the provided checklist when considering submitting an article for publication.

What is the article about?

- A description of innovative practice based on ICN or other guidelines
- A human-interest piece
- An audit of best practice
- An empirical research study
- A theoretical critique
- An opinion piece of international interest
- A literature review.

If the submitted article is research ask the questions:

- Why was the study done?
- What type of study was done?
- Is it primary research (experiment, cohort, case-control, cross-sectional, longitudinal, case report/series)?
- Is it secondary research (overview, systematic review, meta-analysis, decision analysis, guidelines development, economic analysis)?
- Does the article add to what is already in the published literature? If so, what does it add?
- How will the information in the article affect or assist the reader? Does the work matter to clinicians, patients, educators, or policymakers?
- Is the journal for your article submission appropriate for the article topic?

Follow journal guidelines to better ensure acceptance of the work. Journal criteria and journal guidelines are specific to the journal for submission and usually available online or printed in a journal issue.

In general a manuscript for submission should include:

- Title page
- An abstract (brief description of article content; often no more than 250 words)
- Key words used in the article
- Manuscript
- Figures, charts, tables, illustrations
- References

Appendix 8
Example of statements in an ICNP® catalogue on *adherence to treatment*

Nursing diagnosis and outcomes

Ability to manage regime
Adherence to a dietary regime
Denial
Distorted thinking process
Enhanced knowledge
Hopelessness
Impaired family ability to manage regime
Impaired memory
Ineffective coping
Lack of knowledge
Lack of trust in health care provider
Latex allergy
Non-adherence to medication
Low self-esteem
Positive self-image
Readiness for enhanced ability to manage regime

Nursing interventions

Assess attitude to drug management
Assess readiness to learn
Consulting with care provider
Demonstrating subcutaneous injection technique
Determining knowledge
Ensuring continuity of care
Identifying attitude toward care
Identifying obstruction to communication
Maintaining dignity and privacy
Managing drug effect
Managing regime
Promoting medication adherence using pillbox
Reporting status to family member

Teaching about drug
Teaching about managing pain
Teaching about wound care and would healing management
Teaching family about disease
Transporting patient
Verifying allergy

Source: International Council of Nurses. (2005). *International classification for nursing practice (ICNP®)*. Geneva: Author.

Resources

From the International Council of Nurses

These can be ordered at http://www.icn.ch/bookshop.htm or by mail from 3, Place Jean-Marteau, Geneva, 1201, Switzerland. Guidelines are free and most can be downloaded from ICN's web site.

Competencies

ICN framework of competencies for the generalist nurse
This document presents the *ICN framework of competencies for the generalist nurse* at the point of entry to practice. ICN expects that the ICN Framework will be discussed and interpreted by each country, to ensure that they are sufficiently comprehensive and pertinent to a country's health needs and priorities.

ICN framework and core competencies for the family nurse
Reflects the key areas for competency development suggested in the ICN *Family Nurse* monograph and the results of feedback received from an international consultation. The competencies are sufficiently broad to guide the practice of family nursing internationally. At the same time they should be discussed and interpreted in-country, to ensure that they meet national needs.

Education

Guidelines for assessing distance learning programmes
These free guidelines highlight the need to look critically at the feasibility of undertaking this mode of learning, the quality of the programmes available, and the credibility of the provider institution and the award given. They suggest a number of set of screening questions with accompanying statements can be useful in deciding if a programme of study is appropriate for a learner's need and circumstance, is of acceptable quality and offers a recognised credential.

Ethics

Ethics in nursing practice: a guide to ethical decision making. Co-published Blackwell
As well as comprehensive coverage of ethics from diverse cultural and religious perspectives, presents complex ethical issues and real life dilemmas, including those related to HIV/AIDS, abortion, caring for the terminally ill and victims of violence.

Policy and Regulation

Guidelines on shaping effective health policy
These free guidelines address topics such how health policy is made, different approaches to making policy and how nurses and professional organisation can influence policy.

Health policy package (HPP). A guide for policy development
This package is designed to increase the knowledge, skills and abilities of nurses and national nurses associations in the policy process. It is a compilation of ICN's long term experience in developing health policies globally and is divided into four units with specific content, references, resources and activities. It can be used in workshop format or by individuals.

Understanding mutual recognition
This ICN monograph describes the origins and nature of mutual recognition agreements (MRAs) in the context of the globalisation of health care and in what the World Trade Organization calls the movement of natural persons. It focuses on mutual recognition of qualifications, licensing processes and certification requirements that can be used to address issues related to the capacity of professionals to exercise their activities in jurisdictions other than in the country where they were acquired and licensed. It identifies current MRAs affecting nursing, discusses the main features of MRAs and explores important issues, conditions and tasks that lie ahead that help to promote acceptable MRAs.

Practice

Handbook on entrepreneurial practice. Nurses creating opportunities as entrepreneurs and intrapreneurs
This handbook explores what it takes to become a successful nurse entrepreneur or intrapreneur. It has practical advice about roles and services, career planning, building a business and management and financial issues.

Financial management for nurses
An easy-to-use monograph covering *why* and *what* nurses need to know about financial management. It aims to provide a basic knowledge and practical tools for those who are new to this area. It provides useful information for effectively managing resources and budgets, and contributing to key decision-making in today's changing health environment.

Collaborative practice in the 21st century
This ICN monograph explores the definition, elements, characteristics and implications of collaborative practice in health care, in particular offering insights on current and future practice.

ICNP® version 1 – International classification for nursing practice
This new version of the ICNP® classification of nursing phenomena, interventions and outcomes provides a terminology for nursing practice that serves as a unifying framework into which existing nursing vocabularies and classifications can be cross-mapped to enable comparison of nursing data. The package includes the ICNP® Version 1 book and a CD Rom to facilitate teaching and using the ICNP®.

Research

Practical guide for nursing research
This guide is useful for nurses beginning to learn about nursing research. It provides helpful strategies for nurses working to improve the quality of their practice through research.

Ethical guidelines for nursing research
These guidelines refer to the ethical principles for nurses conducting research including guidance on integrity in research, informed consent, data safety and monitoring. Issues related to ethical review boards and misconduct in research are also addressed.

Writing for journals
A revised and simplified edition includes a section on 'hints for authors'. It addresses common delays in publishing and how to avoid them, includes *International Nursing Review* guidelines for authors, a checklist for submitting a manuscript for review and a copyright assignment form.

Guidelines for writing grant proposals
This publication provides a step-by step approach to writing a grant proposal from planning, preparing, writing the proposal and getting funded. It suggests other resources and gives a checklist to use before submitting the grant application.

OTHER RESOURCES

Advanced nursing practice development

Gardner, G., Carryer, J., Dunn, S.V. and Gardner, A. (2004). *Nurse Practitioner Standards Project*. Queensland University of Technology, Australian Nursing Council. This is comprehensive report on the development and progress of the role of nurse practitioners in Australia and New Zealand. It contains an agreed description of the core role of nurse practitioners; an approved set of core competency standards to be applied in Australia and New Zealand; an approved national/trans Tasman standard for education for the accreditation of courses leading to a qualification of nurse practitioners; and a strategy and tools for evaluation and review of the role and standards. Can be ordered from the Australian Nursing and Midwifery Council http://www.anmc.org.au/?event=-1&query=website/ANMC%20Home.html

Jones S., Ross, J. (2003). *Describing your scope of practice: A resource for rural nurses*. Centre for Rural Health: Christchurch, New Zealand.
Although this resource was developed for rural nurses, it describes a process for exploring the dimensions practice in order to describe and define scope of practice. Can be downloaded from www.moh.govt.nz/crh

World Health Organization, Regional Office for the Eastern Mediterranean Region. (In press). *Advanced nursing practice guidelines*. EMRO Technical Publications Series 29, Cairo, Author. These guidelines provide descriptive information, frameworks as well as strategies for consideration and implementation of advanced practice nursing and nurse practitioner roles. Areas covered include titles, definition of advanced practice nursing, scope of practice, characteristics, settings for advanced nursing practice, education: curricula development, standards, regulation and quality assurance.

World Health Organization, Regional Office for the Eastern Mediterranean Region. (In press). *Nurse prescribing guidelines*. Technical Publications Series 28, Cairo, Author. These guidelines were developed to assist countries of the World Health Organization Eastern Mediterranean Region to develop and strengthen nurse prescribing at all levels of health care. They explore the implications of nurse prescribing, offer models of nurse prescribing for deliberation, and provide topics to study when considering introduction of prescriptive authority.

World Health Organization Regional Offices for the Eastern Mediterranean (EMRO) and for Europe (EURO). (2002). *A guide to professional regulation*. EMRO Technical Publication Series, No. 27, Cairo, Author. This joint publication between the Eastern Mediterranean (EMRO) and for European (EURO) WHO Regional Offices aims to strengthen nursing regulation in the two regions and to develop a system to ensure the regulation of nursing practice and education. It provides guidelines on process and content required for institutionalising a comprehensive regulatory system for nursing and midwifery to ensure the highest possible standard of nursing practice and to protect the health and safety of the public. It offers knowledge and information, based on a range of sources and experience, on the processes of creating legislation and establishing effective regulatory systems. Can be obtained from the World Health Organization at http://www.emro.who.int/Publications/Nursing.htm

ICN Accredited Centres for ICNP® Research and Development
German Speaking ICNP® User Group. The German Speaking User Group consists of the three national nursing associations of Austria, Germany and Switzerland and the three national User Groups of these countries. Each partner is represented by one person and a deputy. The role of the three countries' national nurses' associations within the ICNP® Centre is to support the future development and implementation of the ICNP® by using the respective networks and media resources. Contact: Deutscher Berufsberband fuer Pflegeberufe DBfK e.V Geisbergstrasse 39, 10777 Berlin, Germany, icnp@dbfk.de or www.icnp.info

Canberra Hospital and University of Canberra Research Centre for Nursing Practice ICNP® Research & Development Centre
The Australian Centre is located in the Research Centre for Nursing Practice (RCNP), which is a joint facility of Australian Capital Territory (ACT) Health and the University of Canberra. Goals of the RCNP related to ICNP® are to develop the evidence-base for nursing practice, educate and promote the ICNP®, understand the ICNP® framework, facilitate research, and collaborate with the ICN and other ICNP® Research & Development Centres. Contact: Research Centre for Nursing Practice, The Canberra Hospital and the University of Canberra, PX Box 11, Woden, ACT 2606, Australia http://health.act.gov.au/

Chilean Centre for ICNP® Research & Development
The Chilean Centre is located in the Department of Nursing at the University of Concepción. The goals of the ICNP® Centre are to develop a nursing research programme in family nursing, to disseminate ICNP® advances, to incorporate the use of ICNP® in nursing education, and to collaborate in validation of ICNP® terms. Contact: Departamento de Enfermería Facultad de Medicina, Universidad de Concepción, Casilla 160-C, Concepción, CHILE www.udec.cl/

Advanced nursing practice education

Royal College of Nursing. (2002 revised 2005). *Nurse practitioners – an RCN guide to the nurse practitioner role, competencies and programme accreditation.* London, Author.

This RCN document defines the role of the nurse practitioner and sets out the RCN's domains and core competencies for this type of nurse. It also sets out standards, criteria and the type of evidence for RCN accreditation of educational programmes. Can be downloaded from http://www.rcn.org.uk/publications/pdf/NursePractitioners.pdf

National Council for the Professional Development of Nursing and Midwifery. (2002). *Guidelines on the Development of Courses Preparing Nurses & Midwives as Clinical Nurse/Midwife Specialists and Advanced Nurse/Midwife Practitioners.* Dublin, Author. This document deals with programme development, design and evaluation; the curriculum; and programme resources. Can be downloaded from http://www.ncnm.ie/default.asp?V_DOC_ID=906

National Task Force on Quality Nurse Practitioner Education. (2002). *Criteria for evaluation of nurse practitioner programs.* Washington, D.C.: Author. The purpose of this document is to provide a framework for the review of all nurse practitioner educational programs, faculty, curriculum, evaluation, students, organisation and administration, and clinical resources/experiences for all NP educational programs. To obtain copies or to download this document, contact:

American Association of Colleges
One Dupont Circle, NW, Ste. 530
Washington, DC 20036
Tel: (202) 463-6930
Fax: (202) 785-8320
http://www.aacn.nche.edu

National Organization of Nursing
Faculties of Nurse Practitioner
1522 K Street, NW, Ste. 702
Washington, DC 20005
Tel: (202) 289-8044
Fax: (202) 289-8046
http://www.nonpf.com

Uys, L.R. (2004). *Competency in Nursing.* Geneva: World Health Organization. This publication examines the meaning of competence and the benefits of identifying competencies. It gives detailed guidance on the process of deriving competencies and how to formulate competency statements. Finally the use of competencies in nursing is discussed. Can be downloaded from http://rsdesigns.com/extranet/IMG/pdf/Competency_in_Nursing.pdf#search='Competency%20in%20Nursing%20uys'

Advocacy

International HIV/AIDS Alliance. (2002). *Advocacy in action – A toolkit to support NGOs and CBOs responding to HIV/AIDS.* Although this has been developed to support NGOs and community based organisations to advocate for HIV/AIDS it does provide a step-by-step guide to planning and implementing advocacy work and has useful information and advocacy skills-building activities and tools. This can be downloaded from http://www.aidsmap.com/en/docs/4782D096-C740-41A5-AF06-D67C14B46DB8.asp

Sharma, R.R. (Undated). *An introduction to advocacy. Training guide.* Washington, SARA Project – Advocacy Academy for Educational Development.
Introduction to Advocacy Training Guide provides the tools for people to start engaging in the advocacy process, and is thus designed to inform a diverse audience of potential advocates about advocacy and its methods. It aims to teach some basic skills in advocacy; increase the use of available data to inform the advocacy process; give confidence to those who are embarking on advocacy efforts. Can be downloaded from http://pdf.dec.org/pdf_docs/PNABZ919.pdf

Educational Tools

National Council for the Professional Development of Nursing and Midwifery. (2003). *Guidelines for portfolio development for nurses and midwives.* Dublin, Author. Can be downloaded from http://www.ncnm.ie/files/Portfolio%20Guide.pdf. These guidelines address nurses who need to maintain a portfolio. It assists with identifying, reflecting upon and recording the contribution they make to direct and indirect care, and with maintaining records of formal and informal development in a coherent and structured manner. It also provides guidance and information on achieving individual professional goals.

World Health Organization. (1994). *A Guide to good prescribing. A practical Manual.* Geneva, Author. Although the guide is primarily intended for undergraduate medical students who are about to enter the clinical phase of their studies, it has useful material for the advanced nursing practice students seeking to acquire competency in prescribing. It provides step by step guidance to the process of rational prescribing, together with many illustrative examples. It teaches skills that are necessary throughout a clinical career. Can be downloaded from http://whqlibdoc.who.int/hq/1994/WHO_DAP_94.11.pdf

Preceptorship and mentoring

Canadian Nurses Association. (2004). *Achieving excellence in professional practice. A guide to preceptorship and mentorship.* Ottawa: Author. This guide explores the concepts of preceptorship and mentoring as a means to improve performance. It identifies competencies for preceptors and mentors and provides guidelines for setting up preceptorship and mentorship programmes. Can be downloaded from http://www.cna-aiic.ca/CNA/resources/bytype/guides/ default_e.aspx

Queensland Government, Queensland Health. (2001). *Queensland health preceptor program for nursing transitional support. Framework.* Brisbane: Author.
This document explores how organisations can develop and incorporate support mechanisms into their system to support employees who may be entering a new

setting or are new graduates from basic or post-graduate study. It suggests a model to assist employees to cope successfully with the period of time before they are confident and competent in the new range of knowledge, skills and attitudes required. Can be downloaded from http://www.health.qld.gov.au/nursing/docs/11282.PDF

Bibliography from key informants

This bibliography is based on information provided by key informants (personal communication). The authors have tried as much as possible to provide accurate referencing but in some cases complete details were unavailable.

Australia

Australian Nursing Federation. (1997). Advanced Nursing Practice Competencies, Australian Nursing Federation.

Burley, M., Duffy, E., McGrail, M., Siegloff, L. (2002). VRNP2: Victorian Rural Nurse Project – Part 2; Advanced Nursing Practice: Bush Nursing Perspective, Monash University School of Rural Health, Traralgon, Victoria.

Department of Human Services. (1999). Victorian Nurse Practitioner Bulletin, Nurse Policy Branch, August.

Duffy, E. (1999). Advanced Rural Nurse Practitioner, National Healthcare.

Duffy, E., Filmer, M., Rose, P. (2001). 'Quality Care in the Bush' NPPO2-Victorian Nurse Practitioner Project: Phase 2, Nurse Policy Branch, Department of Human Services.

Green, A. & Edmonds, L. (2004). Bridging the gap between the intensive care unit and general wards – the ICU Liaison Nurse. Intensive and Critical Care Nursing, **20**(3), 133–143.

Green, A. (2004). ICU liaison nurse clinical marker project. Australian Nursing Journal, **11**(7), 27–30.

Greene, P., Duffy, E. (2003). Victorian Nurse Practitioner Project – Phase 2; Nurse Practitioner models of Practice: Quality Care in the Bush. Monash University School of Rural Health, Traralgon, Victoria.

Greene, P. & Burley, M., Filmer, M. & Rose, P. (2005). Victorian Nurse Practitioner Project – Phase 2; Clinical Practice Guidelines: Quality Care in the Bush. Monash University School of Rural Health, Moe, Victoria. (In print).

Mahnken, J., Nesbitt, P., Keyzer, D. (1997). The Rural Nurse Practitioner: A pilot project to develop an alternative model of practice. Deakin University, Warrnambool.

NSW Nurses' Association Online. (1999). '40 Nurse Practitioners in Rural NSW in 1999', Newsfront, Professional Roundup, July: 1–3.

Nurses Board of Victoria. (2001). Pre-implementation Report: *The Nurse Practitioner*, Vol. 1, Melbourne, October.

Nursing Branch. (1998). Nurse Practitioner Services in NSW, NSW Health Department, Australia.

Oakes, W. (1999). 40 Nurse Practitioners: Far West leads the way, nursing.aust The Journal @ The New South Wales College of Nursing, Inaugural Issue, November: pp. 1–2.

Offredy, M. (2000). Advanced Nursing Practice: the case of Nurse Practitioners in three Australian States, *Journal of Advanced Nursing*, **31**(2), 274–281.

Siegloff, L., Mathews-Cowey, S. (1995). Nurse Practitioner Project Wilcannia – 1995 Report, Nursing Branch, NSW Health Department, NSW.

Sutton F. & Smith, C. (1995). Advanced nursing practice: new ideas and new perspectives, *Journal of Advanced Nursing*, **21**, 1037–1043.

Transancos, C., Allenby, A., Cameron, J., Haines, H., Green, A., Daniels, J., Flanagan, B., Walker, L., Field, M., & Wapling, A. (2002). The Victorian Nurse Practitioner project. *Australian Nursing Journal*, **10**(3), pp. 19–21.

Whitecross, L. (1999). Collaboration between GPs and nurse practitioners: The overseas experience and lessons for Australia. *Australian Family Physician*, **28**(4), 349–353.

Daniels, J. & Green, A. (2000). Bridging the gap between intensive and ward care. *Nursing Review*, May 2000, 13.

Canada

Alcock, D.S. (1996). The clinical nurse specialist, clinical nurse specialist/nurse practitioner and other titled nurse in Ontario. *Canadian Journal of Nursing Administration*, Jan–Feb, 23–44.

Bryant-Lukosius, D., DiCenso, A. (2004). A framework for the introduction and evaluation of advanced practice nursing roles. *Journal of Advanced Nursing*, **48**(5), 530–540.

Bryant-Lukosius D., DiCenso, A., Browne, G., Pinelli J. (2004). Advanced practice nursing roles: development, implementation and evaluation. *Journal of Advanced Nursing*, **48**(5), 519–529.

Centre for Nursing Studies and the Institute for the Advancement of Public Policy. (2001). The nature of the extended/expanded nursing role in Canada. A project for the advisory committee in health human resources. Centre for Nursing Studies, Newfoundland, Canada. www.cns.nf.ca/research/research. html

DiCenso, A. (2003). Report on the integration of primary health care nurse practitioners into the province of Ontario. www.health.gov.on.ca/english/public/pub/minstry_reports/nurseprac03/nursepract03_mn.html

Dunn, K., Nicklin, W. (1995). The status of advanced practice nursing roles in Canadian teaching hospitals. *Canadian Journal of Nursing Administration*, Jan–Feb, 111–135.

Irvine, D., Sidani, S., Porter, H., O'Brien-Pallas, L., Simpson B., McGillis Hall, L., Graydon, J., DiCenso, A., Redelmeir, D. & Nagel L. (2000). Organizational factors influencing nurse practitioners' role implementation in acute care settings. *Canadian Journal of Nursing Leadership*, **13**(3), 28–35.

Mitchell, A., Watts, J., Whyte, R., Blatz, S., Norman, G., Guyatt, G., Southwell, D., Hunsberger, M., Paes, B. (1991). Evaluation of graduating neonatal nurse practitioners. *Pediatrics*, **88**, 789–794.

Mitchell, A. (1995). Evaluation of an educational program to prepare neonatal nurse practitioners. *Journal of Nursing Education*, **34**(5).

Mitchell, A., Patterson C., Pinelli, J., & Baumann, A. (1995). Assessment of need for nurse practitioner in Ontario. The Quality of Worklife Research Unit, Hamilton, Ontario.

Mitchell, A., DiCenso A., Pinelli, J., Southwell, D. (1996). Introduction and evaluation of an advanced nursing practice role in neonatal intensive care. In *Outcomes of effective management practice*, Kelly, K. (Ed) pp. 171–186, Thousand Oaks: Sage.

Mitchell, A., DiCenso, A. (1996). A controlled trial of nurse practitioners in neonatal intensive care. Pediatrics, **98**(6).

Pinelli, J. (1997). The clinical nurse specialist/nurse practitioner: Oxymoron or match made in heaven. *Canadian Journal of Nursing Administration*, Jan–Feb, 85–110.

Sidani, S., Irvine D., DiCenso A. (2000). Implementation of the primary nurse practitioner role in Ontario. *Canadian Journal of Nursing Leadership*, **13**, 13–19.

Sidani, S., Irvine D., Porter, H., O'Brien-Pallas, L., Simpson, B., McGillis Hall, L., Nagel L., Graydon, J., DiCenso, A., Redelmier, D. (2000). Practice patterns of acute care nurse practitioners. *Canadian Journal of Nursing Leadership*, **13**, 6–12.

Van Soeren, M. (2000). Consortium approach for nurse practitioner education. *Journal of Advanced Nursing*, **32**(4).

Hong Kong

Chang, K.P.K., Wong, K.S.T. (2001). The nurse specialist role in Hong Kong: perceptions of nurse specialists, doctors and staff nurses. *Hong Kong Nursing Journal*, **36**(1), 32–40.

Lum, S. (2004). Development of advanced nursing practice in hospital authority and its role in the era of opportunity. *Hong Kong Nursing Journal*, **40**(2), 13–16.

Twinn, S., Thompson, D.R., Lopez, V., Lee, D.T.F., Shiu, A.T.Y. (2005). Determinants in the development of advanced nursing practice: a case study of primary-care settings in Hong Kong. *Health and Social Care in the Community*, **13**(1), 11–20.

Wong, E.M.L. (2002). Hong Kong accident and emergency nurses' perceived competency in advanced practice and barriers to continuing education. *Hong Kong Nursing Journal*, **38**(2), 7–16.

Wong, F.K.Y. (2004). Advanced nursing practice in Hong Kong: goal-directed, holistic and evidenced-based. *Hong Kong Nursing Journal*, **40**(2), 7–12.

Wong, F.K. (2002). Development of advanced nursing practice in Hong Kong: a celebration of ten years' work. *Hong Kong Nursing Journal*, **38**(3), 25–29.

Macau

Chan, U. (2001). Professional Nursing and Nurse Specialists in Hong Kong and Macau. Revista de Ciencias da Saude de Macau. Macao: Servicos de Saude de Macau.

The Netherlands

Roodbol, P. (2004). Dwaallichten, struikeltochen, tolwegen en zangsporen. Doctoral Dissertation.

New Zealand

Jones, S., Ross, J. (2002). Draft Discussion Document: Career Development Framework for Rural Nurses. National Centre for Rural Health, Dept Public Health & General Practice, Christchurch School of Medicine & Health Sciences, University of Otago.

Jones, S., Ross, J. (2000). A Competency Framework for Developing Rural Nursing. National Centre for Rural Health, Dept Public Health & General Practice, Christchurch School of Medicine & Health Sciences, University of Otago.

Litchfield, M. (2004). *Achieving health in a rural community: A case study of nurse-community partnership*. Hastings, New Zealand: Central Publishing Bureau.

Litchfield, M., Connor, M., Eathorne, T., Laws, M., McCombie, M-L., Smith, S. (1994/2002). Family nurse practice in a nurse case management scheme: An initiative for the New Zealand health reforms. Report of the Wellington Nurse Case Management project funded by the New Zealand Health Reforms Directorate and Department of Health. Wellington: Litchfield Healthcare Associates.

Litchfield, M. (2001). *A framework of complementary models of nursing practice: A study of nursing roles and practice for a new era of healthcare provision in New Zealand*. Christchurch, New Zealand: Centre for Rural Health, Christchurch School of Medicine, University of Otago. www.moh.govt.nz/

Litchfield, M., Ross, J. (2000). The Role of Rural Nurses – National Survey. National Centre for Rural Health, Dept. Public Health & General Practice, Christchurch School of Medicine & Health Sciences, University of Otago.

Ministry of Health. (1998). On Nurse Prescribing in Aged Care and Child Family. Health Consultation Document, Wellington: Author.

Ministry of Health. (1997). Draft Discussion Document: Extending Limited Prescribing Rights to Registered Nurses, Wellington: Author.

Ministry of Health. (2002). *Nurse Practitioners in New Zealand.* Wellington: Author.

National Centre for Rural Health. (2003). An Educational Programme to Foster Collaboration for Rural Teams. Dept Public Health & General Practice, Christchurch School of Medicine & Health Sciences, University of Otago.

New Zealand Government. (2001). Designated Prescriber: Nurses Practising in Aged Care and Child Family Health. Medicines Regulations 2001/230.

Nursing Council of New Zealand. (2001). *Framework for post-registration nursing education.* Wellington: Author.

Nursing Council of New Zealand. (2002a). *The Nurse Practitioner: Responding to Health Needs in New Zealand*, 3rd Edition, Wellington: Author.

Nursing Council of New Zealand. (2002b). *Nurse Practitioner Endorsement: Guidelines for Applicants.* Wellington: Author.

Ross, J., Jones, S. (2002). Scope of Practice Tool for Rural Nurses, National Centre for Rural Health, Dept Public Health & General Practice, Christchurch School of Medicine & Health Sciences, University of Otago.

Ross, J. (2001). Dimensions of Team Effectiveness in Rural Health Services. National Centre for Rural Health, Dept. Public Health & General Practice, Christchurch School of Medicine & Health Sciences, University of Otago.

Ross, J. (2000). The National Role of Rural Nursing Project – Executive Summary. National Centre for Rural Health, Dept Public Health & General Practice, Christchurch School of Medicine & Health Sciences, University of Otago.

Ross, J. (1996). Rural Practice Nurse Skills Project (SRHA). Centre for Rural Health, Dept Public Health & General Practice, Christchurch School of Medicine & Health Sciences, University of Otago, (available from author).

Spence, D. (2004). Advancing Nursing Practice through postgraduate nursing education, Part 1 and 2. *Nursing Praxis*, Vol. 20, 2/3.

Thailand

Langkarpint, P. (2004). The development of advanced practice nursing in Thailand: Passage and process. Doctoral dissertation for the University of Hull, UK.

United Kingdom

Evans, C., Rogers, S., McGraw, C., Battle, G., Furniss, L. (2004). Using consensus methods to establish multidisciplinary perspectives on research priorities for primary care. *Primary Health Care Research and Development*, **5**(1), 52–59(8).

Long, A., McCann, S., McKnight, A., Bradley, T. (2004). Has the introduction of nurse practitioners changed the working patterns of primary care teams?:

A qualitative study. *Primary Health Care Research and Development*, **5**(1), 28–39(12).

Myers P., Lenci B., Sheldon M. (1997). A nurse practitioner as the first point of contact for urgent medical problems in a general practice setting. *Family Practice*, **14**(6), 492–497.

Venning, P., Durie, A., Roland, M., Roberts, C., Leese, B. (2000). Randomised controlled trial comparing cost effectiveness of general practitioners and nurse practitioners in primary care. *British Medical Journal*, **320**(7241), 1048–1053.

Venning, P., Roland, M.O. (1995). New opportunities in practice nursing: roles matter more than titles. *British Medical Journal*, **311**(6996), 3–13.

Switzerland

De Geest, S., Hasemann, W., Kesselring, A. (2005). Delirium-Management am Universitätsspital Basel – ein Beispiel angewandter Pflegewissenschaft (Delirium management at the University Hospital of Basel. As an example of applied nursing science). *Managed Care.*

Müller-Frölich, C., Conca-Zeller. (2005). Pflegewissenschaft als Partner der klinischen Praxis (Nursing science as partner of clinical practice) (Editorial). *Managed Care*, **6**, 6–8.

Spirig, R., Nicca, D., Werder, V., Voggensperger, J., Unger, M. (2004). The Advanced Nursing Practice Team as a Model for Caregiving in HIV/AIDS. *Journal of the Association of Nurses in AIDS Care JANAC*, **15**(3), 47–55.

Spirig, R., De Geest, S. (2004). Advanced Nursing Practice lohnt sich! (Advanced Nursing Practice is worthwhile) (Editorial). *Pflege: Die wissenschaftliche Zeitschrift für Pflegeberufe*, **17**, 233–236.

Spirig, R., Kesselring, A., Werder, V., Voggensperger, J., Unger, M., Bischofberger, I., Nicca, D., Battegay, M., De Geest, S. (2002). Entwicklung und Etablierung einer erweiterten und vertieften HIV/Aids Pflegepraxis (Developing and establishing an expanded and more comprehensive HIV/AIDS nursing practice). *Pflege: Die wissenschaftliche Zeitschrift für Pflegeberufe*, **15**, 293–299.

Spirig, R., Petry, H., Kesselring, A., De Geest, S. (2001). Visionen und Perspektiven für die Zukunft: Die Pflege als Beruf im Gesundheitswesen der Deutschschweiz (Vision and Perspectives for the Future: The nursing profession in the Swiss German Health Care System). *Pflege: Die wissenschaftliche Zeitschrift für Pflegeberufe*, **14**(3), 141–151.

Ullmann-Bremi, A., Spirig, R., Gehring, T.M., Gobet, R. (2004). Outcomes and experiences of caring for families with children with cleft lip and palate at the Children's Hospital of Zurich. *Pflege*, **17**, 243–251.

Ullmann-Bremi, A., Spirig, R., Ullmann, S. (2004). A method combination for Advanced Nursing Practice projects. *Pflege*, **17**, 262–269.

Glossary

Accreditation is a process of review and approval by which an institution, programme or specific service is granted a time-limited recognition of having met certain established standards beyond those that are minimally acceptable.

ICN Definition 1997, updated 2004

Advocacy is an action directed at changing the policies, positions and programmes of any type of institution.

Sharma (undated)

Advanced nursing practice distinguishes a higher level of practice from that of the generalist nurse based on an advanced level of critical thinking, decision-making and increased accountability in practice.

Adapted from Rolfe, G., Fulbrook, P. (1998)

Advanced practice nurse: a registered nurse who has acquired the expert knowledge base, complex decision-making skills and clinical competencies for expanded practice, the characteristics of which are shaped by the context and/or country in which s/he is credentialed to practice. A masters degree is recommended for entry level.

ICN Definition, 2002

Approval is a process of review by which an institution and/or programme is judged to have met the prescribed minimum standards set by the appropriate standards body. Approval is distinguished from accreditation in that the approval process is usually not voluntary, and the standards-setting body is usually governmental.

ICN Definition, 1997, updated 2004

Assessment is a systematic procedure for collecting qualitative and quantitative data to describe progress, practice and achievement.

ICN Definition, 1997

Autonomous practice is the authorised performance of the activities that are included in the advanced practice nurse's legitimate scope of practice, active professional responsibility and accountability for the outcomes of those activities. In some

210

cases of independent practice, the advanced practice nurse serves as a first contact provider or entry point into the healthcare delivery system and has the responsibility for her/his own patient case-load. Sometimes independent and autonomous are used interchangeably.

ICN Definition, 2005

Bridging programme: a programme of study designed to provide individuals with skills and knowledge required for entry into an occupation, or a higher-level educational institution. It supplements learning outside of a jurisdiction, or at another institution and may include workplace training, occupation-specific skills and language training.

Adapted from CICIC, 2003

Capacity building (or development) is the process by which individuals, organisations, institutions and societies develop abilities (individually and collectively) to perform functions, solve problems.

United Nations Development Programme UNDP, 1997

Career mobility is the movement of nurses to more advanced levels to different areas of nursing practice or to positions in which different functions predominate.

ICN, 1993

Career development in nursing is a process underpinned by lifelong learning and risk taking, by which a nurse incorporates personal values, aptitudes and interests to shape a career path that supports personal growth and professional development and enhances the contribution of the nursing profession to society. Career development enriches current performance and builds a nurse's capacity to take advantage of, or create, future opportunities.

ICN Credentialing Forum, 2002

Certification is a voluntary time-limited process by which a non-governmental organisation within a profession or specialty grants recognition of competence to an individual who has met pre-established eligibility requirements and standards.

ICN Definition, 2004

Collaborative practice is an integrated approach to delivering services. Health providers function as colleagues and are grounded by common care goals, supported by shared decision-making, and nourished by a climate of mutual respect, trust and support. Effective communication and clear definitions of roles and responsibilities are integral to success.

ICN Definition, 2004 (Schober & McKay)

Competence is the effective application of a combination of knowledge, skill and judgement demonstrated by an individual in daily practice or job performance.

ICN Definition, 1997 (Styles & Affara), updated 2004

In nursing definitions, there is wide-ranging agreement that, in the performance of nursing roles to the standards required in employment, competence reflects the following: knowledge, understanding and judgement; a range of skills – cognitive, technical or psychomotor and interpersonal; and a range of personal attributes and attitudes.

Continuing competence is the ongoing ability to integrate and apply the knowledge, skills, judgement, and personal attributes required to practice safely, competently and ethically in a designated role and setting.

Adapted from CNA, 2004

Continuing education refers to the whole range of learning experiences, from the time of initial qualification until retirement, designed to enrich the nurse's contributions to quality health care and her/his pursuit of professional career goals.

ICN Definition, 1997 (Styles & Affara), updated 2004

Continuing professional development refers to the establishment of higher levels of competence in the range of knowledge, skills and abilities needed to perform duties or support interventions, be they in clinical practice, management, education, research, regulation or policy making.

ICN Definition, 1999

Credential: documented evidence of having met predetermined standards. It communicates to employers, payers, and consumers what to expect from a 'credentialed' person, specialist, course or programme of study, institution of higher education, hospital or health service, or health care product, technology, or device. Credentials may be periodically renewed as a means of assuring continued quality and they may be withdrawn when standards of competence or behaviour are no longer met. Degree, diplomas, certificates, licences are examples of credentials.

ICN Definition, 1997 (Styles & Affara), updated, 2004

Credentialing is a term applied to processes used to designate that an individual, programme, institution or product have met established standards set by an agent (governmental or non-governmental) recognised as qualified to carry out this task. The standards may be minimal and mandatory or above the minimum and voluntary. Licensure, registration, accreditation, approval, certification, recognition or endorsement may be used to describe different credentialing processes.

ICN Definition, ICN, 1997 (Styles & Affara)

Criteria are descriptive statements which are measurable and which reflect the intent of a standard in terms of performance, behaviour or circumstance.

ICN Definition, 1997

Curriculum is a statement of the intended aims and objectives, content, experiences, outcomes and processes of an educational programme including a description of the structure (entry requirements, length and organisation of the programme, and assessment system) and of expected methods of learning, teaching, feedback and supervision.

Adapted from Postgraduate Medical Curriculum for General Practice

Equivalence refers to the process where, although two differing standards or procedures remain intact, they are treated as if they are the same because, in theory, they produce the same or similar result.

Adapted from TACD, 2000

Generalist nurse: has the scope of preparation for practice that enables her/him to have the capacity and authority to practise competently primary, secondary, and tertiary (care for chronic, long-term illness) health care in all settings and branches of nursing.

ICN Definition, 1986

Guidelines are interpretative statements, which serve to extend and clarify meaning, but are not intended as an absolute standard.

ICN Definition, 1997

Human resource development (HRD) refers to functions involved in planning, managing and supporting the professional development of the health workforce within a health system, both at the strategic and policy levels. HRD aims at getting 'the right people with the right skills and motivation in the right place at the right time'.

World Bank, 2005

Human resources planning is a process of creating an adequate organisational environment and ensuring that the personnel perform adequately using strategies to identify and achieve the optimal number, mix and distribution of personnel in a cost-effective manner.

World Bank, 2005

Licensure is the process, sanctioned by the law, of granting exclusive power or privilege to persons meeting established standards, which allows them to engage in a given occupation or profession, and to use a specific title.

ICN Definition 1997, updated 2004

Mandatory regulation is usually applied when the authority for regulation is governmental usually through a statute and approval for practice is legally required. Standards are usually set at the minimum required for public protection.

ICN Definition, 1997

Mentoring is a voluntary, mutually beneficial and long-term relationship where an experienced and knowledgeable leader (mentor) supports the maturation of a less experienced nurse with leadership potential (mentee).

Canadian Nurses Association, 2004

Mutual recognition is a vehicle for regulatory co-operation, and it may be based on harmonisation, equivalence, or external criteria such as the host country's standards or other mutually agreed standards, or international standards. In a mutual recognition agreement, two or more parties agree to recognise and accept all, or selected, aspects of each other's regulatory results because they are harmonised or judged to be equivalent, or because they satisfy other agreed-upon external criteria. Results may include assessment outcomes, qualifications, standards, rules, titles, and quality assurance system standards.

Adapted from TACD, 2000

Nurse entrepreneur: a proprietor of a business that offers nursing services of direct care, educational, research, administrative or consultative nature. The nurse is directly accountable to the client, to whom, or on the behalf of whom, nursing services are provided.

ICN, 2004

Portfolio: a professional portfolio is an organised collection of documents demonstrating education, experience, knowledge, competencies and capabilities in an area of advanced nursing practice, and shows the depth and scope of practice undertaken by the applicant, as well as a capacity to analyse and reflect on practice.

Adapted from NCNZ, 2002

Nurse practitioner (see advanced practice nurse): a registered nurse who has acquired the expert knowledge base, complex decision-making skills and clinical competencies for expanded practice, the characteristics of which are shaped by the context and/or country in which s/he is credentialed to practice. A masters degree is recommended for entry level.

ICN Definition, 2002

Preceptorship is a frequently employed teaching and learning method using nurses as clinical role models. It is a formal, one-to-one relationship of pre-determined length, between an experienced nurse (preceptor) and a novice (preceptee) designed to assist the novice in successfully adjusting to a new role. The novice may be a student or an already practising nurse moving into a new role, domain or setting.

Canadian Nurses Association, 2004

Professional regulation is all the legitimate and appropriate means – governmental, professional, private, and individual – whereby order, identity, consistency and control are brought to the profession. The profession and its members are defined; the scope of practice is determined; standards of education and of ethical and competent practice are set; and systems of accountability are established through these means. Also may be called governance.

ICN Definition, Styles & Affara for ICN, 1997

Protocol: a detailed written template or procedure for the treatments of a specific health problem.

Adapted from Hanson, 2005

Recognition is the formal acceptance of an institution, programme or service by another institution or public authority. It may also mean the acceptance of knowledge, skills, or formal qualifications of an individual and the granting of advanced standing or credit.

Adapted from CICIC, 2003

Regulatory body: the formal organisation designated by a statute or an authorised governmental agency to implement the regulatory forms and processes whereby order, consistency and control are brought to the profession and its practice.

ICN Definition, 1997

Scope of practice is the range of roles, functions, responsibilities and activities, which a registered/licensed professional is educated for, competent in, and is authorised to perform. It defines the accountability and limits of practice.

ICN Definition 1997 (Styles & Affara), updated 2004

Skill-mix: can refer to the mix of posts in the establishment; the mix of employees in a post; the combination of skills available at a specific time. Alternatively, it may refer to the combinations of activities that comprise each role, rather than the combination of different job titles. 'Skill-mix' and 'nursing-staff-mix' are often used interchangeably in the literature.

Adapted from O'Brien-Pallas et al., 2005

Self-regulation (self-governance) is the governance of nurses and nursing by nurses in the public interest.

ICN Definition, 1997 (Styles & Affara)

Specialist nurse: a nurse prepared beyond the level of a nurse generalist, and authorised to practise as a specialist with expertise in a specified field of the nursing.

ICN Definition, 1989, updated 2004

Stakeholders are persons, groups or institutions with interests in a project, policy, proposed action, or programme which may ultimately affect them, either positively (beneficiaries) or negatively.

Adapted from Overseas Development Administration, 1995

Standard: the desirable and achievable level of performance against which actual practice is compared.

ICN Definition, 1989

Statutory regulation is regulation mandated by a law, act, decree or statute.

ICN Definition, 1997 (Styles & Affara)

Telehealth is the delivery of health care and health care related services across time, and distance barriers through the use of telecommunications technologies.

ICN Definition, 2000 (Milholland)

Telenursing is the term used to denote the use of telecommunication services to deliver nursing services.

ICN Definition, 2000 (Milholland)

Validation is the process of making judgements about professional, vocational and academic programmes, which may lead to a recognised award. This recognition will include meeting criteria reflected in the rules and regulations of the participating bodies.

ICN Definition, 1997

Voluntary regulation is conducted by an authority external to the government. The credential or qualification thus earned is not legally required for practice or the service to be rendered.

ICN Definition, 1997 (Styles & Affara)

References

Canadian Information Centre for International Credentials (CICIC). (2003). *Guide to terminology in usage in field of credentials recognition and mobility*, Ontario, Author.

Canadian Nurses Association. (2000). *A national framework for continuing competence programs for registered nurses*, Ottawa, Author.

Canadian Nurses Association. (2004). *Achieving excellence in professional practice. A guide to preceptorship and mentorship*, Ottawa, Author.

Hanson, C.M. (2005). *Understanding Regulatory, Legal, and Credentialing Requirements*. In Hamric, A.B., Spross, J.A. and Hanson, C.M. *Advanced Practice Nursing. An Integrative Approach*, 3rd Edition, pp. 781–808, St Louis, Elsevier Saunders.

International Council of Nurses. (1987). *Definition of nurse generalist*. Working definition approved by the Council of National Representatives.

International Council of Nurses. (1989). *Definition of nurse specialist*. Approved by the Council of National Representatives, Author.

International Council of Nurses. (1997). *An approval system for schools of nursing. Guidelines*. Geneva, Author.

International Council of Nurses. (1999). *The ICN system for awarding international continuing nursing education credits. Introduction*. Geneva, Author.

International Council of Nurses. (2002). *Definition and characteristics for nurse practitioner/advanced practice nursing roles*, Geneva, Author.

International Council of Nurses. (2004). *Guidelines on the nurse entre/intrapreneur providing nursing services.* Geneva, Author.

International Council of Nurses. (2005). *The scope of practice, standards and competencies of the advanced practice nurse.* Working ICN Document.

Milholland, D.K. (2000). *Telehealth and telenursing: Nursing and technology advance together.* [Monograph 4]. ICN; Author.

O'Brien-Pallas L., Duffield C., Murphy G.T., Birch S. & Meyer R. (2005). *Nursing workforce planning: mapping the policy trail.* Geneva, International Council of Nurses.

Overseas Development Administration. (1995). *Guidance note on how to do stakeholder analysis of aid projects and programmes.* Retrieved 22 December, 2005 from http://www.euforic.org/gb/stake1.htm

Postgraduate Medical Curriculum for General Practice. *What is curriculum?* Retrieved 16, November, 2005 from http://www.gpcurriculum.co.uk/theory/definition_curriculum.htm

Rolfe, G., Fulbrook, P. (Eds) (1998). *Advanced nursing practice.* Oxford: Butterworth-Heinemann.

Schober, M. & McKay, N. (2004). *Collaborative practice in the 21st century.* Geneva, International Council of Nurses.

Sharma, R.R. (Undated). *An introduction to advocacy. Training guide.* Washington, SARA Project–Advocacy Academy for Educational Development.

Styles, M.M. & Affara, F.A. (1997). *ICN on regulation: Towards a 21st century model.* Geneva, ICN.

Trans Atlantic Consumer Dialogue (TACD). (2000). *Briefing paper on mutual recognition agreements (MRAs).* Retrieved 10 October, 2005 from http://www.tacd.org/cgi-bin/db.cgi?page=view&config=admin/docs.cfg&id=193

United Nations Development Programme. (1997). Capacity development. Technical advisory paper II. In Capacity Development Resource Book. New York, Author. Retrieved October 20, 2006 from http://magnet.undp.org/cdrb/Default.htm

World Bank. (2005). *Health systems development: Glossary.* Retrieved 21 October, 2005 from http://www.worldbank.org/

World Health Organization. (2002). Human resources, national health systems. Shaping the agenda for action. Final report. Geneva, Author.

Index